Nursing Ethics

Ian E. Thompson BA(Hons) PhD
Senior Educationist, Scottish Health Education Group

Kath M. Melia BNurs(Manc) PhD SRN NDN HV
Lecturer, Department of Nursing Studies, University of Edinburgh

Kenneth M. Boyd MA BD PhD
Scottish Director, Institute of Medical Ethics

SECOND EDITION

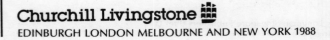

Churchill Livingstone

EDINBURGH LONDON MELBOURNE AND NEW YORK 1988

CHURCHILL LIVINGSTONE
Medical Division of Longman Group UK Limited

Distributed in the United States of America by Churchill Livingstone Inc., 1560 Broadway, New York, N.Y. 10036, and by associated companies, branches and representatives throughout the world.

First edition 1983
Second edition 1988

ISBN 0 443 03458 3

British Library Cataloguing in Publication Data
Thompson, Ian E.
  Nursing ethics. — 2nd ed.
  1. Medicine. Nursing. Ethical aspects
  I. Title II. Melia, Kath M. III. Boyd,
  Kenneth M.
  174'.2

Library of Congress Cataloging in Publication Data
Thompson, Ian E.
  Nursing ethics.
  Bibliography: p.
  Includes index.
  1. Nursing ethics. I. Melia, Kath M. II. Boyd,
Kenneth M. III. Title. [DNLM: 1. Ethics, Nursing.
WY 85 T472n]
  RT85.T476   1988   174'.2   88-6138

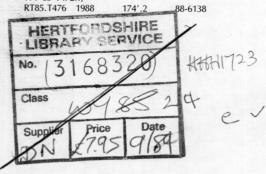

Produced by Longman Singapore Publishers (Pte) Ltd.
Printed in Singapore.

Preface

This book is a basic guide to nursing ethics. Nursing ethics today is a subject of study in its own right. It can no longer be regarded simply as a branch of medical ethics or of ethics in general; nor can it be regarded simply as a matter of passing on hints and tips about manners and morals. In 1900, the American nurse Isabel Hampton Robb published a book with the same title as this one. In it she stated that ethics 'teaches men the practice of duties of human life and the reasons for what they do and for what they should leave undone' (Robb 1915). Statements of this kind reflected the philosophies and popular confidence of the time that ethics was largely about doing your duty and that your duty was largely obvious. As far as nurses were concerned, it was summed up in the demand for 'implicit, unquestioning obedience' (Robb 1915) and in the requirements of conventional respectability. Today things are not so simple. The social and professional hierarchies within which modern nursing was established no longer seem part of an eternal order: nurses, while recognising a proper division of labour between themselves, medicine and the other health care occupations, no longer take the view that it is 'ours not to reason why'; and the study of ethics, in a plural, multicultural society, now supplies at least as many unsolvable moral dilemmas as clear ethical imperatives.

Changes of this kind, together with developments in medical science and technology, and evidence, this century, that even members of professions with high ideals can sometimes act unethically, has greatly increased professional and public interest in medical and nursing ethics. Interest in nursing ethics in now apparent in nursing conferences and the nursing press, as well as in the time increasingly being set aside for teaching the subject in nursing curricula. All of this is an indication that in ethics, as in other aspects of nursing practice, research and teaching, Florence Nightingale's dictum is again relevant: 'What cruel mistakes are sometimes made by benevolent men and women in matters of business about which they can know nothing and think they know a great deal' (Skeet 1980).

In relation to nursing ethics, this advice points to the need for those with practical knowledge of nursing's real moral dilemmas now to engage in common study with those from other disciplines, including those with some skill in asking pertinent questions and exploring their implications. If nursing ethics is to be taught or studied well, an interprofessional approach is necessary.

This book is largely the result of attempts to put this interprofessional approach into practice. The collaboration, in its authorship, of a philosopher, a nurse and a theologian arose out of their earlier co-operation in the work of the Edinburgh Medical Group and in nursing ethics teaching, particularly at Queen Margaret College, Edinburgh. The authors are particularly grateful to the staff and students of that college for stimulating their thinking and providing a great variety of helpful insights on the matters discussed in the book. They are grateful also to several groups of nurses, and nurse tutors, who met to advise on its contents, both when the book was first mooted and later, when this revised edition was in view. In planning and revising the book the authors were fortunate in having the assistance of Dr Alison Tierney, Dr Alison Kitson and Mr Jim Brown, who, while not responsible for its defects and shortcomings, made many helpful suggestions about its form and content. The staff of Churchill Livingstone also must be thanked for their patience and practical assistance.

This book is about moral issues in nursing and the ethics of nursing care. How to deal in real life with moral problems and moral dilemmas, of course, is not something anyone can learn from a book. It is a matter, rather, of action and reflection on action, of making mistakes and learning to live with the knowledge that we shall probably make mistakes in the future. The most that this or any book on the subject can do is to set out and criticise arguments for and against the moral alternatives which face us. A book of this kind, in other words, is simply an extension of what happens when we discuss our moral choices or dilemmas with other people.

Thinking about everyday moral problems or dilemmas we almost inevitably begin by seeing these from our own point of view; but if we listen attentively to other people involved in the situation, or to an impartial friend, we often begin to see other sides to the question which, in turn, affect what we feel we ought to do. So in discussing moral choices generally, or problems and dilemmas in particular, there usually are more sides to the question and more kinds of relevant moral arguments than we begin by recognising. The aim of a book of this kind, therefore, is to identify and criticise some of these different arguments. But having done that, the book has not provided us with 'answers'. Learning to see our everyday moral choices through the eyes of others involved, or of an impartial adviser, may make us sympathetic or vulnerable to their points of view: but it does not make our choice for us.

Similarly, when we study moral questions, we become aware of the variety of arguments for and against different alternatives, their strengths and weaknesses: but in the end this usually leaves us with more questions than answers, and the choice, in practice, remains our own. The advantage of studying the arguments, in other words, is much the same as the advantage of listening to other people: it expands our intellectual horizons in the hope that this will make us less self-centred and short-sighted: but it does not make our choices for us, nor does it make choosing any easier.

While collaborating in the preparation of the book, each of the authors has adopted a different but complementary approach to the subject. Dr Boyd contributed Chapter 1, which introduces the subject of ethics, moral choice and values in very general terms, related as much to common everyday experience as to nursing in particular. Dr Melia, in the next two chapters, writing from the standpoint of a nurse and sociologist, sets the moral issues to be considered in the context of the experience of becoming and being a nurse in the world of patient care and professional organisation. Dr Thompson contributed the remaining chapters. These represent the application of the methods of moral philosophy to a range of questions in nursing ethics. Chapters 4 and 5 deal with power-sharing and fundamental values, and key moral issues in nursing ethics. Chapters 6, 7 and 8 cover a number of typical cases, suggested by nurses themselves, selected to illustrate three different kinds of areas in which moral problems and dilemmas may be encountered in nursing; in the direct nurse–patient relationship, in management of groups of patients, and in the wider relationships of nurses and society. The final two chapters deal with moral decision-making and the relevance of moral philosophy or ethical theory to nursing ethics.

The different approaches represented by the authors, it is hoped, may help to indicate the breadth of the area with which nursing ethics is concerned, as well as the depth of the issues which it raises. It is intended to be of interest to all nurses, from student nurses to senior managers, but some sections may be of more interest to some readers than to others. For example, the first five chapters will be of general interest to all nurses, Chapters 6 and 7 may be of more relevance to nurses directly involved in patient care, while Chapter 8 may be of more interest to managers. The final chapters will be particularly helpful to readers wishing to study ethics more systematically, as they examine in greater depth theoretical questions involved in the book's discussion of moral issues. In general, the authors hope that this book will be found useful not only for private study by nurses and others but also in the increasing number of ethics seminars and courses of the kind out of which it arose.

REFERENCES

Robb I H 1915 Nursing Ethics. Cleveland, p. 15, 57
Skeet M 1980 Nightingale F: Notes on Nursing. Churchill Livingstone, Edinburgh, p 111

Contents

Moral issues in nursing and the ethics of nursing care

1.1 What do we mean by ethics?

Nursing is only one area of life in which we face moral choices, and while it has many special features which we will consider later, it also has much in common with the rest of our moral experience. By way of introduction, therefore, we will begin by defining some terms and discussing what we mean by them in the context of this book: 'ethics' and 'morals', 'moral problems' and 'moral dilemmas', 'moral choice', and 'moral values'. We will discuss these first in the context of ordinary life, noting how perceptions of moral issues and choices are related to the ways in which moral values may change over time.

What, in the first place, do we mean by ethics and morals? These terms originally meant much the same thing, 'ethics' coming from Greek and 'morals' from its Latin equivalent. Both words referred to the general area of the rights and wrongs, in theory and practice, of human behaviour. In everyday usage moral and ethical can still be used more or less interchangeably, but a distinction has grown up between the two terms in more formal usage. Morals (and also morality) now tends to refer to the standards of behaviour actually held or followed by individuals and groups, while ethics refers to the science or study of morals — an activity, in the academic context, also often called moral philosophy.

This distinction, however, is complicated by three popular ways of using the words. 'Ethics' can also be used to refer to the morals or morality of certain groups, such as the professions, and sometimes to the morals or morality of individuals: the implication behind this usage is that the morals or morality involved either have been codified or carefully worked out, or that they are in some sense high-minded. Associated with this idea of high-mindedness is the second popular use — that of both 'moral' and 'ethical' as terms of approval, the opposite of 'immoral' or 'unethical'. The third popular use seems to derive from the idea of ethics as the impartial study or science of morals. This use is seen when 'ethics' and 'ethical' seem to be preferred to 'morals' and 'morality' because the latter are thought of as having some connection either with sex on the one hand or with religious dogmatism on the other; 'ethics' and 'ethical', by contrast, are thought of as involving something more cerebral and objective. However, there is no substantial reason for these associations of ideas, which are largely a matter of preference, only slightly if at all more justifiable than the habit of preferring 'ethical' to 'moral' apparently for no better reason than that it sounds more impressive (Downie 1980).

1.2 Moral problems and moral dilemmas

Given this background of different usages then, what do we mean by moral problems and moral dilemmas? Both terms confront us with choices which involve our beliefs and feelings about what we fundamentally regard as good or right — our moral values or moral principles. We distinguish between moral problems and moral dilemmas because there is a tendency in popular discussion in the media and the nursing press to refer indiscriminately to all difficult situations requiring moral decisions as dilemmas. There is also a risk that people, confronted with a so-called 'dilemma', will avoid taking responsibility for decisions. Whereas there may be things that can be done, if someone is prepared to take responsibility.

In everyday life we often deal with *problems* requiring a

moral decision. These may involve completely new and unfamiliar situations, but more often we are dealing with day-to-day problems which tend to recur. Past experience of similar situations equips us to face specific problems with some knowledge of how to deal with them, however painful or difficult the choices may be. Because 'problems', clearly defined and understood, usually have solutions, or possible solutions, they are not of the same kind as moral dilemmas — although we may need courage to tackle them. A *dilemma* is a choice, of whatever kind, between two equally unsatisfactory alternatives. Not all dilemmas are *moral* dilemmas; some dilemmas are the result of not knowing the best means, in theory or practice, to an agreed end. Nor are all moral choices moral dilemmas, since in many cases we may well know what we ought to do and the question is whether we will do it. What makes the choice a moral dilemma, rather, is the fact that it involves conflict between moral principles — what we believe we ought to do — and moral values — what we think of as, or feel to be, fundamentally good or important and thus value as something we would act upon. We feel, in other words, that certain moral values or principles would make us adopt the one alternative, but also that others would make us adopt the other alternative, but we cannot adopt both. Choosing the one alternative means not only not choosing the other, but actually going against what the value or principle it represents would have us do.

1.3 Moral dilemmas in everyday life

Moral dilemmas arise from time to time in the lives of most people. For example:

A student has promised her classmates that she will write up their group project, which must be handed in to their tutor the next morning. Just after she has started to write, her closest friend telephones in great distress, wanting to see her right away because her fiance has just broken off their engagement. A few days later the student is approached on a snowy street by an emaciated beggar who asks her for the price of a cup of tea. The student can easily afford to give him this, but the beggar clearly has alcohol on his breath and it is only 10 o'clock in the morning. Later in the day the student meets her married sister who is worried about her 14-year-old daughter. The daughter has asked if she can go to the next town tomorrow with a girlfriend to see a new film and come back on the late train. She says that the other girl's parents have agreed, but her mother is unable to contact them and is not sure that her daughter has told her the whole story.

These experiences are moral dilemmas because a choice between conflicting moral values or principles seems to be involved in each case. The first experience involves, on the one hand, the moral principle that we should keep our promises: on this side of the dilemma there is also the moral value of being a good or dutiful student. On the other side there is the moral value of being a good friend; there is also the moral principle that we should help others in need. The conflict here is not between different things the student *wants* to do (her best friend or the group project may each in their own way be tiresome and the alternative a welcome excuse) but between different things which she feels she *ought* to do.

Meeting the beggar, the student may want to give him the money — perhaps to get him out of the way, perhaps to make herself feel virtuous. But she may also feel that she ought not to, because it would not be in his interest to continue drinking himself to death. On the other hand, she may not want to give him the money — perhaps because she is afraid the beggar may recognise her and pester her again. She may also feel that she ought to give it, because as another adult the beggar has a right to decide what is best for himself — and because one ought to help others in need.

The sister's dilemma, too, involves the right of another person to decide what is best for themselves, but in this case is complicated because the other person is a child. If teenagers are to become responsible adults, parents have to learn to trust them to be responsible, even if this means letting them make their own mistakes. On the other hand, some mistakes can have serious consequences, and parents have a responsibility also to protect their children. If the mother values responsibility, that value will exert considerable moral pressure on both sides of her dilemma.

1.4 Information, communication and choice

The above examples all seem to be genuine unresolvable

moral dilemmas. But certain facts might emerge which could question this. The student might have failed to read a notice from the tutor postponing the project deadline for a week. The beggar might have been at a crucial stage in voluntary psychiatric treatment for alcoholism. The other girl's parents might have agreed to her going to the cinema on the condition that one set of parents collected the two girls by car. In each case this vital information, if it had come to light, might well have resolved — or dissolved — the respective dilemma. In the case of the project this would be for obvious reasons. In that of the beggar, the student might be able to argue that because his psychiatric treatment was voluntary her refusal of money was supporting his own prior decision about what was best for himself. As far as the girls were concerned, the information might allow the mother to negotiate an agreed compromise with her daughter about the degree of responsibility appropriate to the circumstances.

Possibilities of this kind illustrate the importance, when facing moral dilemmas in everyday life, of adequate information and good communication. Quite often, what appears to be a moral dilemma is the result of a breakdown in, or the absence of, relevant communication between different people. This is certainly true of some areas of interprofessional and professional–patient communication, with which we will be concerned later.

If a nurse does not know what a doctor has told a dying patient, she may not be sure whether to give a truthful reply to the patient's question about what is happening to him. When the bed of a patient awaiting discharge is urgently needed for another patient, and the nursing staff fail to discover, for example, that a relative has just arrived at home to look after the first patient: the misconception that this patient has nowhere to go could create an avoidable moral dilemma about priorities. So sometimes, especially when the same kind of moral dilemma regularly occurs, rather than agonising over each dilemma, it may be worth asking whether institutional or personal networks of communication cannot be improved in some appropriate way, either by some organisational means or by those involved cultivating a greater degree of tact or ingenuity.

1.5 Making moral decisions

Improvements in communication clearly have a part to play in avoiding certain unnecessary moral dilemmas. On the other hand, there may be a temptation, particularly among practically minded people, to overestimate what can be achieved in this way. The student's dilemma, we might say, could have been avoided either if the college had had a better system of informing students, or if the student herself had cultivated the habit of checking notice-boards more carefully. Her sister's dilemma, too, might have been avoided had she worked harder, over a longer period of time, at communicating with her daughter. Even the dilemma involving the beggar might have been avoided if the student, on meeting him, had talked to him and elicited the vital information. A way round the moral dilemma can be found, in each of these suggestions, just as, often enough, it can be found in everyday life. On the other hand, there are many situations in everyday life when no such way exists; and even when it does, and the acute moral dilemma can be avoided, the fact of moral choice and moral conflict remains.

To illustrate this fact, consider the examples again. Meeting the beggar, the student might have started to talk with him and he might just possibly have given her the vital information. But in thus delaying any decision about whether to give him the money until she had more information, the student was already acting in a way which — at that time, with the information she had — went against what on one side of her dilemma she felt she ought to do; it went against, that is, another adult's right to decide what was best for him. Her decision to seek more information in this case was not a morally neutral matter: she had come down on one side of the dilemma and made a moral choice.

Prior moral choice might equally have been involved in any means by which the other two dilemmas could have been avoided. A better system of informing students might have been possible for the college only at the cost of choosing not to spend its limited resources on, say, library facilities or student amenities. Again, in cultivating the habit of checking notice-boards more regularly the student might have been opting for a general style of living which gave greater priority to the demands of work than to the demands of friendship.

Here, too, moral choices would have been involved, as they would have been in the sister's decision to spend more time with her daughter — which might well have been at the expense of time spent on her own work or with her husband.

Even when ways exist of avoiding acute, painful or recurrent moral dilemmas, then, this does not mean that moral choices are not being made. Such choices may have been made over a long period of time, as the characters of individuals, relationships or institutions were being formed. But the succession of small choices made every day by everyone, individually or collectively, is no less significant than the large choice which an acute or painful moral dilemma confronts us with. In this sense, everything that we do to some purpose can be seen, in principle at least, as the result of some moral choice made by us as individuals or as part of present or past society.

What all this suggests is that moral dilemmas, which we may reasonably wish to avoid in everyday life, can nevertheless play a useful part in our understanding of the moral dimension of our experience. The point about moral dilemmas is that they demonstrate, more dramatically than other aspects of our experience do, the inescapability of moral choice in everyday life.

A moral dilemma brings into sharper focus the moral values and principles which, even when they conflict with one another, matter to us because of our previous moral choices, many of which have been everyday choices and relatively unconsidered but which, cumulatively, have gone to make up what we may call our moral character. Confronted by a moral dilemma, the fact that we recognise it as such challenges us also to recognise the strength of our conflicting values, and in making — or not making — a moral choice, to adopt, change or reinforce the nature of our moral character. In studying moral issues, then, while it is reasonable enough to look — as we would in everyday life — for ways round or out of the dilemma, it is also useful to consider the dilemma on the assumption that there are no such ways, and to ask, if that is the case, which option we would choose and how we would defend our choice in the light of the values involved. When we have begun to do that, it might be added, we have begun to study ethics.

1.6 Shared and changing values

In what has been written so far, moral values have been discussed mainly in terms of the values of individuals. But values, of course, are something we share. This can be seen in the fact that morals and politics are not distinct activities but part of a continuum. People, it is true, sometimes talk about politics as if it were only a matter of power for power's sake; but while power clearly is of importance in politics generally and to some politicians in particular, politics is also concerned with ideals and social goals, and values play an important part in political as well as moral dilemmas. Some of the earliest moral philosophers, Aristotle in 384 BC for example, considered that the study of ethics was part of the study of politics; and clearly enough the purposes, values and principles we have as individuals cannot be properly studied in isolation from those of the society and culture which have made us what we are (Thomson 1976).

The fact of shared, as well as individual, values is of obvious importance in considering practical moral issues in nursing and the ethics of nursing care in general. Some of the ways in which becoming a nurse may create shared values among members of the profession, and also create conflicts with the individual's values, will be discussed in Chapter 2, and the relationship between moral rules and roles will be mentioned in Chapters 3 and 9. In Chapters 4 and 5 the relationship between power and values, values and fundamental principles, and values in health care will be discussed further. In this discussion, in the broader context of everyday moral choice, however, it may be worth asking how our shared values have been changing, and what effect this may be having on our contemporary moral decision-making.

One of the major changes which seems to have taken place in our society during the last century is a shift from general public agreement about moral values to much greater variety of expressed moral opinion and tolerance of diversity. Not everyone 100 years ago, of course, agreed about what was morally right and wrong, nor today is society without consensus on some moral issues. But the variety of moral viewpoints which it is acceptable to express and possible to justify in public does seem to have become greater. This situation of *moral pluralism* may well be one reason why we are particularly aware today of moral conflicts and dilemmas. How we view this situation will depend on our moral presuppositions: some of us will see it as symptomatic of moral liberation, others of moral decay. The truth is probably, as usual, more complex and, because we are living through it, largely hidden from us. On the basis of what has happened to societies in the past, one way of interpreting what is happening now may be by comparing it with the transition from childhood to adolescence.

An obvious aspect of this comparison is the way in which many people today look back nostalgically to the lost moral certainties of the past. This nostalgia is reminiscent of what, in retrospect, seems so attractive about childhood — its security and particularly the certainty of childhood ideas. Grandmother is a saint, father can do anything, our family's ways are the best ways, the others' are rather odd. The pain, but also the excitement, of adolescence lies in discovering that things are really much more complicated and often not what they had seemed. Grandmother can be an emotional tyrant, father has not conquered the world, other families' ways and moral standards may be as good as, if not better than, ours. The change experienced in adolescence, in other words, is from a world in which things are morally black or white to one in which we discover an infinite variety of moral shades of grey. In this situation we are faced with two major temptations. One is to deny that the shades of grey exist, possibly by adopting a new black and white morality supplied by some dogmatic moral, religious or political ideology. The dangers of this are those of moral short-sightedness about the complexity of real-life decision-making, and moral insensitivity towards those with different convictions. The other temptation is to accept the infinite variety of moral shades of grey and to say that they are all the same. The dangers here are those of moral indifference and moral indecisiveness.

One way of understanding what has been happening to morality in our society, then, is to compare it with this transition from the moral certainties of childhood to the uncertainties, temptations and dangers of adolescence. Similar changes have taken place in the past, when individuals or societies have experienced the transition from tribal or village life to the life of large cosmopolitan cities. In the tribe or village, morality was a matter of shared fixed conventions which gave people considerable security — but at the price, often, of hypocrisy, guilt, and even open cruelty towards those who deviated from the moral norm. The shift to city life, where people from different origins with different moral views lived together, made it difficult to maintain the old black and white certainties, revealed the moral shades of grey and exposed individuals and society to the adolescent's temptation to question all values or take refuge in dogmatism. In our time, something of the same kind seems to have been happening to society generally through experiences of war, the growth of travel, international communications, the mass media and public education. These developments have made more people that ever before aware of the variety of moral viewpoints which it is possible to hold, and consequently of the difficulty, in the face of this, of maintaining that any one traditional moral viewpoint is right or the best. Here we face the same risks, of *moral dogmatism* — the uncritical acceptance of a particular moral position as infallible — or *moral relativism* — the view that any moral position is as good as another.

Against this background, one particular value which has fallen in public esteem is that of paternalism and the principle that 'father knows best'. This shift is associated with greater respect for the value of self-determination and the related idea of human rights — especially the rights of women and of minorities. Involved in this change also is an emphasis on the individual which favours such values as self-expression rather than self-sacrifice, tolerance rather than conformity, and flexibility rather than strict obedience to moral rules. Changes of this kind seem to be reflected today in changing attitudes within nursing, traditionally a female, obedient, self-sacrificing and sometimes rigid profession. These changing attitudes focus on questions about the authority of the traditionally male profession of medicine, the separate identity of nursing as a profession in its own right and the need for more flexible ways of providing care. Changing values also seem to be reflected in contemporary concern for such things as the patient's right to know and the right to choice and self-determination in health care.

This account of changing attitudes and moral values in our

society is merely one impression of what has been happening; and it can be immediately conceded that the changes suggested are far from universal. That such changes are far from universal is, in fact, part of the point, since a major difficulty in moral decision-making today is the unpredictability of the values held by other people. Frequently, it is not possible when making difficult moral choices to rely on an appeal to values which, in the past, might have been expected to command general support. In nursing, for example, there is still considerable reluctance to go on strike. But this reluctance cannot be relied upon as much as in the past; and it is likely to be defended only in some cases by an appeal to the traditional values of duty and obedience. In other cases the defence is more likely to be in terms of the value of care or concern for patients, or even of the profession's self-interest where strikes are thought to be counterproductive.

As this example suggests, the variety of moral values which different people hold today is a matter of practical concern as well as of theoretical interest. Conflict between moral values exists not only on either side of the moral dilemmas confronting individuals, but also within society and between different societies. The great divisions in today's world are not only about material issues of power, wealth and poverty, but also about which moral values should have priority in the ordering of society. Should liberty be put first as in Western societies, or equality as in Socialism, or the law of God as in resurgent Islam? Moral conflicts of this kind, clearly, can spill over into social, economic and even physical conflict within societies as well as between them. While political bargaining can play some part in the attempt to reconcile different interests, the purposes, ideals and values which move individuals and societies to action must also be taken into account if the harmful consequences of conflict are to be avoided.

In seeking to avoid these harmful consequences, it is important to remember that moral conflict in itself is not bad. Indeed it is only through moral conflict that society can resist the temptations of individual moral dogmatism and moral relativism, and thus remain responsive to the variety of moral values in personal and communal life which makes life fully human. To resist these temptations and at the same time avoid the harmful consequences of conflict is not easy, and perhaps not even possible, unless individuals and societies have some way of communicating with one another which helps each to understand the importance of the other's moral values without thereby diminishing the importance of their own. In human life there are many ways of establishing such communication, ranging from marriage to international diplomacy. But one useful way, we would suggest in the present context, is through the kind of informed and reasoned public debate about moral issues which we undertake in the study of ethics. Such debate provides a framework within which people can communicate with one another about the values and principles which move them to action; a framework within which they can give one another reasons why they believe these values and principles to be important, can offer and listen to reasonable criticism and can, on occasion, find ways of establishing public consensus about the rights and wrongs of particular conflicts. In an area such as health care, at a time of increasing recourse to the courts and to political bargaining, ethics would seem to have a particularly useful contribution to make.

Of course, this is not to suggest that we all need to become philosophers any more that we are all able to be saints. Nor is it to suggest that someone who has mastered the technical language of ethics is necessarily thereby a better person or even someone better able to resolve moral difficulties in practice — indeed the opposite is often the case. But it does suggest that to make ourselves vulnerable to, and critical of, the ethical arguments and moral sentiments of others is a more creative and constructive way of responding to the moral complexity and conflicts of our time than by retreating either into moral dogmatism or into moral relativism. Vulnerability is probably the key word here. Moral dogmatism and moral relativism are each in their own way attempts to be invulnerable to moral conflict, by pretending either to have no doubts or that none of it matters. The point we have been trying to make in this introductory chapter and which, we hope, will be apparent in the following chapters is that moral conflict does matter and that, in practice, we can rarely be entirely sure that our actions have always been right or for the best. This is particularly true in the field of health care, where professionals are frequently required to act quickly and decisively in matters affecting the vital interests of patients. To ask such professionals also to be vulnerable to such knowledge, and thus to the pain and guilt it may involve, is no doubt hard. But it is only in accepting such vulnerability, perhaps, that any of us escapes from moral adolescence into precarious adulthood.

REFERENCES AND FURTHER READING

. Beauchamp T L, Childress J F 1979 Principles of biomedical ethics. Oxford University Press, Oxford.
Downie R S 1980 Ethics, morals and moral philosophy. Journal of Medical Ethics 6: 33–36
Downie R S, Calman K C 1987 Healthy respect: Ethics in health care. Faber, London.
Gillon R 1986 Philosophical medical ethics. Wiley, Chichester.
MacIntyre A 1967 A short history of ethics. Routledge & Kegan Paul, London.
Thomson J A K (trans) 1976 The ethics of Aristotle, revised edn. Penguin Books, Harmondsworth, bk 1.

2

Becoming and being a nurse

2.1 On entering the nursing profession

The decision to become a nurse may well be made in much the same way as a decision to become anything else — an architect, say, or secretary or a market gardener. In the case of nursing, however, the word 'become' is more apt than it is for many other professions. Becoming a nurse is not simply a matter of learning particular knowledge and skills, or adopting forms of behaviour appropriate to particular contexts. It is also a matter of assimilating the attitudes and values of the nursing profession in a way which can profoundly influence the thinking, personality and lifestyle of the individual concerned. In other words, being a good nurse not only demands theoretical knowledge and practical expertise, but also growth in moral experience or practical wisdom. This combination of knowledgeable skill and acquired moral responsibility is what Aristotle called 'virtue'. Virtue and vice are defined by him as habitual forms of action which have become second nature. Although nurses should never stop learning, being a nurse means having the confidence to act wisely on the basis of acquired clinical and moral experience.

In this chapter we shall discuss some aspects of what it means to be and become a nurse. To do this, some ideas from sociology will be drawn upon in order to set the individual nurse making moral decisions in some kind of context, a social organisational context which shapes and influences those decisions. The purely sociological outlook which sees the world in terms of roles, processes of socialisation, social organisation and social structure may not be helpful at a personal level, but it provides us with some understanding of where individuals come from and what factors are likely to influence or constrain their actions. On the other hand, traditional ethics may be said to be too individualistic if we are attempting to examine the activities of a professional group providing a public service. We aim to strike a balance between the two and to look at the possible ways in which nurses might contemplate the moral aspects of their work. At an individual level we might think that nurses are motivated mostly by an ethic of caring. When student nurses are asked at interview why they want to become nurses, a common response is that they want to 'care for people'. However, when we look at the way in which nursing care is delivered in public health services, it becomes clear that professional nursing has to be organised on principles which are rather less individualistic than the notion of simply caring for patients. Hospital-based and community nursing require competent and efficient services organised to provide equal access and fairness in the distribution of health care resources for all in need.

We will consider first the difference between professional and lay nursing, together with some of the moral conflicts which arise in the sphere of the nurse's relationship with other health professionals.

2.2 Nursing, lay and professional

Those entering the nursing profession often do not realise that their chosen sphere of work will involve difficult decisions which may call into question their own personal convictions and values. Today, of course, the lay conception of nursing involves some appreciation of the difficulties and conflicts faced by health professionals. Discussion in newspapers and on television has made the general public aware of ethical issues in health care. Nevertheless, it is probably true to say that nurses are not generally thought to have moral responsibilities or to face conflicts of such magnitude as those encountered by doctors. Doctors are highly special-ised and skilled, and in the popular view they are often seen to be dealing daily with matters of life and death. The lay view of nursing, by contrast, is probably less dramatic. Nursing, moreover, is something which lay people themselves do: it is, after all, carried out by members of the family at home and by untrained, as well as trained, personnel in hospitals. The lay view of nursing, in other words, may make it difficult for newcomers to the profession to appreciate the responsibili-ties and complexities and hence the moral conflicts which they will encounter.

In order to appreciate these responsibilities, complexities and conflicts, it is necessary to look a little further at the simi-larities and differences between lay and professional nursing. Looking after a sick relative at home involves doing things for the patient which he cannot do for himself, preventing the patient from undertaking anything which will impede his recovery, and administering any treatment or medication which has been prescribed. Leaving aside some of the tech-nicalities of modern hospital care and allowing that professionals have a greater degree of relevant information and resources, these are essentially the same activities a qual-ified nurse would undertake either in the home or in hospital (Henderson 1966). In terms of what nursing involves at a prac-tical level, therefore, it is difficult to establish how the care given by a lay person differs from that provided by nurses. Nevertheless, the two types of care do differ, in at least three fundamental ways. First, nurses undertake their work not on the basis solely of duty, altruism or necessity, but on a contractual basis. Professional nurses look after patients in return for payment and, in the case of trainee nurses, to gain their professional qualifications (Campbell 1985). Secondly, nurses and patients are not normally involved in one another's lives in any sphere other than the nurse–patient relationship. Lay nursing, by contrast, usually takes place within the context of a family or of friendship, thus involving a different kind of carer–patient relationship. Thirdly, the nurse and patient in the professional setting may well come from different backgrounds and thus not share the same outlook, culture, values and expectations.

2.3 The transition from lay to professional

During the transition, or the socialisation process, the learner discovers and adopts the professional approach to nursing in terms of practical skills and of attitudes and values. The latter may cause particular difficulties, either across generations or between individuals. But such difficulties arise against the background of a lifetime of family differences and agreed ways of negotiating them. The needs of the individual, rather than the demands of a large organisation, are the pivot of decision-making. In professional nursing, by contrast, there exist not only institutional pressures but also the need for co-existence between the values of an individual and of a profession. The risk of conflict between these personal and professional values is at its height during the early years of training, when the new recruit has not yet been socialised to the extent of having adopted for herself the values of the profession.

The risk of such conflict is particularly acute in nursing because, while socialisation may be incomplete, the transition at a functional level has to happen quickly. Learners spend a short time at a college of nursing absorbing some of the basic tenets of nursing care, and they have a chance to visit the hospital wards to see these in practice. Then one day a student finds herself standing in a ward, a patient calls 'Nurse' — and means her. At this functional level, the student abandons lay status almost overnight. What, though, of the deeper adjustments to be made? When does the student feel like a nurse?

It is in such experiences of being and yet still becoming a nurse that the learners meet their first conflicts. On the one hand, they have to confront their own personal feelings and reactions to the situations in which they find themselves and, on the other hand, the values and attitudes of the professional group they have joined. For example:

A learner is being shown round her new ward by the staff nurse. It is a geriatric ward, and clearly a busy one. She has been told that after a quick tour she is to work with a third-year student and that by such an arrangement they should 'get straight by lunchtime'.
Halfway down the ward there is a lady in her eighties, sitting by her bed. As they approach, she asks the learner to tell her the time and what is for lunch, and while speaking she secures a firm grip on the

learner's uniform skirt. The staff nurse announces loudly that Mrs B is always asking the same questions because she is demented and has a grossly impaired memory. She gives no indication as to how the newcomer is to extricate herself from the situation while conveying clearly the message that she is to be followed down to the dayroom to complete the tour of the ward.

In this situation the personal moral code of the learner might dictate that she should stay and talk to the patient. At this level it matters little to the learner whether the patient is demented: she is another human being who has started a conversation with her. All the learner's past experience of life tells her to provide an answer and to conduct the conversation as she might any other. However, within the context of nursing, this old lady's request for information has been re-interpreted as the product of her dementia and as such can and should be legitimately ignored so that the 'real' work of nurses may progress.

2.4 Socialisation and sensitivity

A situation such as the above demonstrates the initial sensitivity which newcomers to the nursing profession possess while at the same time indicating how, once the professional approach to the work is adopted, this initial sensitivity becomes threatened. This desensitising process is to a large extent synonymous with the socialisation process. Much of the difficulty involved in 'becoming' a nurse is bound up with feelings of inadequacy and inability to cope with the reactions the introduction to nursing provokes in an individual. The newcomer has no stock of responses to these new encounters such as with patients in pain, dependent sick adults, young cancer sufferers and the victims of road traffic accidents. Past experience, values and personal moral convictions might yield a set of emotional responses to these new encounters, but they do not provide any prescription for action or reaction. The new recruits thus soon adopt the ways of nursing they see around them. This can be said to be due, in part, to their lack of alternatives and, in part, to the efficiency of the socialisation process.

One of the consequences of an efficient socialisation process is the appearance of well-ordered professional behaviour, with everyone assuming an air of confidence and security in the knowledge that their behaviour is in line with the 'professional way'. This makes life even more difficult for the newcomers, as they tend to feel that everyone is coping except themselves. Learners might well think that they are the only ones to feel shocked by some of the sights they meet: for example, the soon to be taken-for-granted sight of so much nakedness, the lack of privacy and a seemingly matter-of-fact approach to human suffering. These feelings of shock, revulsion, or simply of inadequacy are further evidence of the naivety and sensitivity of the new recruits to nursing. Yet the concurrent suggestion, often made by learners themselves, that they should not register any such feelings, reveals the fact that already they have some notion of the professional attitude towards such feelings. It is more probably these early observations which make trainee nurses aware that they are weighing up nursing against their own standards. The first sightings of a surgical wound, a colostomy, an amputation or a demented patient, and above all the experience of caring for dying patients can profoundly shock the newly arrived learner. It is in terms of such encounters that the junior nurse confronts personal feelings and values with the professional values of nursing.

The speed with which the new recruits adopt the prevailing mode of nursing has both advantages and disadvantages. On the positive side it affords the learners some fairly immediate ways of coming to terms with what they see, and of finding a way of functioning. By looking around them they see what others do, others who are seemingly coping and are not distressed by what they see, and follow suit. Indeed the newcomer learns how to carry out nursing work with more confidence and competence and so the socialisation process serves the common good, as well as enabling nurses to cope with crises and emotionally stressful situations. The disadvantage in the newcomer's so readily adopting the 'professional' approach to nursing is, as has already been suggested, that it puts at risk the initial sensitivity, where personal moral values dominated. An example might be the way in which the toilet needs of patients on a geriatric ward are met. Trainee nurses might well be initially offended by the idea of several old ladies being supplied with commodes en masse and with little privacy. As the weeks go by, however, they will become accustomed to such practices, even if they do not come fully to accept them.

Because newcomers are at a loss as to how to behave when faced with patients, they will often feel silly and incompetent. Their major concern might well be to find some way of meeting the expectations of the trained staff. In so doing, learners can be well aware that they are compromising their own value systems in the way that they feel they must behave towards patients. For example, hospital meal-times are often rushed affairs, where the main nursing objective might well appear to a newcomer to be to serve meals and collect in plates, empty or otherwise, in the shortest space of time. Learners, given the task of feeding a reluctant patient, are often placed in a situation where they feel obliged to hurry the patient in order to satisfy the expectations of the staff. At the same time, learners feel a natural response of sympathy for the patient and, following their own instincts, might be disinclined to hurry him or her or, if he is very reluctant, even to feed him. Again, there is a conflict between the preferred individual behaviour of the learner and that of the experienced nurse.

2.5 The organisation of nursing

The distinction between lay and professional approaches to nursing can be elaborated in terms of the organisation of nursing in order to provide some further understanding of the conflicts which the professional style of nursing presents. Lay nursing is essentially organised on an individual basis — one patient with one or more carers who know one another. The way in which nursing is carried out is thus constrained, for the most part, only by the needs of this small group of people. The lay activity of nursing is able to follow a pattern based on a set of values normally worked out over a long period of time. Professional nursing, on the other hand, is usually carried out on a larger scale and involves people who do not know each other. Even taking account of the moves towards individualised care introduced into nursing under various banners — team nursing, patient allocation, nursing process — the fact remains that professional nursing is organisationally oriented and operates along the lines of routine approaches to care. Routines are less accommodating for individuals with regard to their personal needs or particular beliefs and values. This lack of emphasis upon the individual is true for both patients and nurses. It should perhaps be noted that colleges of nursing teach recruits a form of nursing which lays stress upon the individual. The patient is the central focus and the learners are taught to plan care according to individual needs (Melia 1984). This denies the reality of the routinised approach to nursing found on many wards.

2.6 Roles and individuals

Professional nursing within an organisation relies upon the notion of role rather than individual. That is to say there are several roles, for example nurse, patient, relative, doctor and so forth into which individuals are placed. Their expected behaviour within the organisation is detemined by the role and not by the person. This arrangement means that a certain uniformity is introduced into the system, for along with each role goes a set of expectations, responsibility and privileges. In practical terms, this means that certain forms of behaviour can be expected of the incumbents of different roles: the nurse is expected to care for patients in a way such as the whole body of professional nurses would recognise and deem fit. Similarly, a patient, whoever he is, is expected to follow the dictates of his carers, to be grateful for their care and to do his best to comply with the treatment (Parsons 1970). In this way an organisation such as a hospital can function without every individual having to start from first principles with everyone he meets. The rules of behaviour are laid down, and adherence to role expectation is the key to the success of such an organisation.

There remains, one problem. That people adopt roles is only one side of the coin: they also retain their individuality. The person who adopts the role of a nurse takes on the legal and moral obligations of nursing as defined by statute and the profession. But at the same time nurses do not relinquish their individual character with their personal beliefs and values. It is the co-existence of personal values and professional values which presents many practical and ethical problems for nurses. The nurse may ask, himself or herself, 'What ought I to do, feel or think?' Emmet (1966) explored the question of what 'is' and what 'ought' to be and suggested how one determines what the 'ought' might look like. Much of what people think they ought to do is governed by how they see their roles. Nurses as individuals may want to act in one particular way, yet in their role of nurse they feel that they ought to act differently.

2.7 Routine and compromise

The mainstay of the professional approach to nursing is routine. Nursing care can be reduced to a set of routines designed to meet the needs of a group of patients. Patients have individual needs, but in their role of 'patient' they can be added to other patients and have their overall needs provided along organised professional nursing lines rather than lay individual lines. In this way the nursing care of a group of patients can be conceived of as a workload to be got through. One of the most efficient ways to do this is to divide the care into a series of tasks and share them, and incidentally, the patients, among the nurses. This practice faces learners with a further kind of conflict — to decide whether they should hold on to the principles of 'good' nursing they have been taught and proceed along the individualised lines of care put forward by the college, or simply join in the routine care being practised. In the event they have little choice, since being junior nurses they will invariably do as they are told. However, this does not remove the conflict, since learners have the added problem of living with their consciences if they feel that they have compromised judgement and acted against the interests of patients.

Unfortunately, at this early stage, while students are still able to see with new eyes what goes on in nursing, they are also preoccupied with becoming nurses, that is with behaving as other nurses do. By the time the recruits have become accustomed to the work and are less frightened and perplexed by the realities of nursing they have probably also lost some of that initial innocence. To return again to an earlier example, new nurses are often struck by the dehumanising aspects of hospital care. (Melia 1987). Patients appear to have little control over their life in hospital; there is greatly reduced privacy and intimate procedures and issues are often treated seemingly lightly. The new nurse's perspective in all of this is in some ways closer to the lay perspective of the patient than it is to that of the professional nurse. Still in the process of transition from the lay to the professional perspective they can empathise with the patient. At this early stage, however, the learner is in no real position to influence the style of care given. By the time learners reach a stage when they feel that they might exert their own views and carry out their nursing according to their own judgements, there is a danger that the sights which initially offended and provoked a desire to respond in a way which was not congruent with professional values, are now commonplace. This may not necessarily mean that the learner has lost touch with the lay approach to nursing and its attendant personal values. It may mean that the actual consideration of the ethical implications of seemingly straightforward nursing work must now be a deliberate and critical activity, rather than a spontaneous reaction.

The process of becoming a nurse is in some ways similar to that of becoming a patient. The loss of a certain amount of identity, taking on a generalised role and behaving accordingly, are experiences common to nurses and patients. The student has a uniform, the patient nightwear; decisions about day-to-day living have been taken from the person and placed in the hands of the organisation, for example mealtimes, off-duty for the nurse, waking and sleeping times for the patient. New nurses often feel that they are in a rigid hierarchy which relies upon rank and punitive measures rather than rationality and reason. Their freedom to act and question what they see is sometimes restricted. This leaves many of the conflicts of personal and professional values unresolved.

The process of 'becoming' a nurse, then, requires the recruit to adopt an approach to nursing consistent with that adopted by the profession as a whole. The socialisation process is by and large an efficient one, since few lay people have the resources to cope with the demands of nursing at an individual level, and newcomers tend to opt for the security which goes with adopting the profession's values.

However, the socialisation process is not perfect; if it were, nurses would behave in an entirely predictable and non-individualistic way. The adoption of professional nursing values can only go so far. There may always be some residual tension between the individual and his or her personal values and the expectations which go with the role of the nurse who operates according to professional ethical mores. There are clearly positive advantages to be gained from adopting the nursing profession's modes of behaviour, rather than relying upon individual moral judgements. Each individual nurse must then cope with any discontinuities which may exist between personal values and those of the profession. Such discontinuities do not cease with qualification. Up to this point we have studied two kinds of moral question facing the learner. How can personal and professional values be reconciled? And how can the individual nurse practise 'good' nursing in the face of accepted compromise? Having become a nurse, the individual finds that these questions, although sometimes now easier to avoid, do not go away.

2.8 Relationships and feelings

One area in which questions continue to arise is that of building up relationships with patients. From their earliest days in college, nurses are made aware of the importance of building good relationships between themselves and patients. If patients are to gain the maximum benefit from nursing care, they must trust the nurse who gives it. The same advice is sometimes given in a different way by saying that patients must be considered as persons (Ramsey 1970). How does the total patient care approach work out in practice? It suggests that the nurse should become intimately acquainted with a number of patients. But these patients will be people towards whom the nurse is likely to have the normal range of human feelings. And alongside the advice to build relationships with patients as people, the nurse will also constantly hear the advice, 'Do not become too involved'.

In formal terms, the advice to treat patients as persons involves respect for the individual patient's rights as well as for what the nurse or the health care system may consider to be the patient's interests. The socialisation process lays much emphasis upon acting in a professional manner and not getting too involved with patients. Such considerations tend to detract from the central issue, which has to be the respect for patient's rights. (This is more fully discussed in Chapter 6.)

However, in terms of the nurse's feelings about actual people, there may be difficulties and conflicts. The nurse may well feel much more sympathy for, say, a young leukaemic patient of the same age than for an elderly demented patient at the end of his life — or, for whatever reasons, it may be the other way around. In the everyday life of nurses outside their sphere of work, the fact that there are some people they take to, some they dislike, and many about whom they have no strong feelings is something they may take for granted on the assumption that it takes all sorts to make a world. But when much the same mixture of people arrive as patients, the demands of building good relationships and treating them as persons are much more difficult. Clearly, nurses cannot be forced to like people to whom they may feel an aversion, any more than the patients with similar feelings towards nurses can be forced to like them. Under these circumstances the nurse may adopt the Hippocratic maxim, 'First, do no harm', to ensure that an instinctive dislike is not reflected in overt attitudes. Nurses may also be grateful for the positive feelings which make it easier to treat certain patients as persons. In the end, the nurse will still remain prey to a range of different feelings towards other people, and these feelings will have a potential for harm as well as good. Furthermore, these feelings are never entirely suppressed or removed by the process of socialisation, so it is important that they are recognised.

The fact that nurses have perfectly natural feelings of like and dislike for particular patients, and that these feelings can do both good and harm, clearly lies behind the advice not to become involved. How far each nurse heeds this advice, and how far they find it incompatible with building good relationships with patients as persons, must ultimately be a matter for individual judgement. But judgement is not formed in isolation, and there are factors in the interaction of nurses with seniors, peers and patients, which may exert an unrecognised influence. One such factor is the effect on nurse–patient relationships of the practice of labelling patients.

2.9 Labelling patients

The theory of labelling comes from the sociology of deviance and has to do with our attitudes to people with attributes which we do not consider normal (Lemert 1951, Becker 1963). These attributes may relate to their health problems, physical or mental pathology, or to their physical appearance, personality type or other particulars. Sociological analysis of diagnostic labelling in medicine and its significance in the clinical management and social control of patients emphasises both the privileges and obligations of the 'patient' within the 'sick role' (Freidson 1970, Parsons 1970). A diagnosis of renal failure, schizophrenia or alcohol-dependent syndrome has benefits for patients, in legitimating their access to resources for care or treatment and allowing them to adopt the 'sick' role and then get time off work, claim sickness benefits/insurance and so on. However, even these medical labels are potentially stigmatising and impose obligations on patients to co-operate in the prescribed forms of treatment even if these are inconvenient or distressing. In this context, however, we wish to examine the way nurses label patients, and the significance this has for nurse–patient relationships (Bond & Bond 1986). For example, nurses may refer to patients as 'difficult' or 'unco-operative' or to their behaviour in terms of 'He won't help himself', 'Just trying it on', 'Doesn't want to get well', and so forth. In this way, behaviour which makes the nurses' work more difficult is deemed to be deviant. By implication, this makes the nurse the innocent party in any encounter — a position strengthened by drawing upon the support of colleagues in the use of the label. For example:

A patient who is used to working shifts does not settle early to sleep and prefers either to watch late-night television or to read. The nurse whose job is to follow hospital policy and turn the ward lights out by 10.30 p.m. finds this patient difficult to cope with. Because the patient feels strongly about staying up, he makes a great fuss each night and wins his fight to watch the late television film. The nurse, when handing over shifts, reports that he is 'being awkward' again. In the patient's terms, this simply means going to bed at his usual time.

When nurses use this technique of labelling, then, it serves to legitimise the feelings that individual nurses may have towards a patient. Nurses can then think in terms which make, say their own impatience with a patient seem not their own fault. In the case, for example, of a patient who is making slow progress from a stroke, the nurses may have applied the label of 'Doesn't try', which in turn shields the nurse who tries to get the patient dressed in the morning from her own feelings of frustration or even anger. When labelling is used in large institutions such as hospitals, more-over, the labelled behaviour can take on the character of a stereotype. The term 'awkward patient', for example, is then more simply a description of one individual, it conjures up for the nurse a whole set of forms of behaviour expected from any patient thus labelled. To some extent, of course, such labelling and stereotyping is an inevitable part of social interaction. But the patient's vulnerability and dependence on the nursing staff mean that it has more far-reaching effects in his case than in everyday life. It is therefore particularly important that the nurse should be aware of what she is doing in applying or agreeing to a label. Is the label really accurate? Or is it simply a way of defending or excusing herself at the patient's expense?

Not all labels are of the kind described so far. A patient might be labelled as 'dependent', 'a child', 'dying' or 'mentally retarded', and labels of this kind can have some functional significance. They are not necessarily labels which the patient himself would agree with: and again, even cate-gory labels of this kind can be used in ways which are less in the interests of the patient than in that of the professional's own self-justification. There are, however, a number of category labels whose use has achieved a degree of consensus among health carers, and in discussing the moral questions we are concerned with further, it may be useful to look at one or two of these in greater detail.

2.10 Difficult and unpopular patients

Patients can be labelled as 'difficult' for a variety of reasons. A demanding elderly patient, a private patient who treats nursing staff as paid servants or a non-compliant patient all tend to attract this description. The old lady who rings her bell every time the nurse leaves the room is clearly as entitled to the services of the nurse as the lady in the next room who hardly ever asks for anything. Nevertheless the nurse is likely to feel annoyed with the old lady who wastes nurses' time and may often be tempted to use minor sanctions against her, or to resort to delaying tactics. Any attempt to justify this understandable kind of response, however, must overcome the objection that the nurse, being the stronger party in the relationship, has a greater responsibility to act in a just or fair way towards the weaker. Treating patients as people, in other words, involves respecting their rights — even when they seem to abuse them.

The nurse's problem in handling personal feelings is more complicated when conflicting demands arise. The nurse may feel antagonistic to an alcoholic or 'overdose' patient, who seems to have brought his troubles upon himself. But when a young girl, say, who has taken an overdose is brought in to a casualty department — followed within minutes by the victims of a serious road accident — the nurses who are left to look after the girl may well feel that they could be better employed working with the more 'deserving' accident victims. Similar problems may arise among nurses working in gynaecological wards' where those having terminations may be nursed alongside infertile women who desperately want children. In situations of this kind, judgemental labelling may be a strong temptation for those whose personal moral values create antagonism. Unpopular patients may consequently be at some risk of having their psychological if not physical needs undervalued. The principle of justice is important here, for not only is the patient in danger of having his rights to proper physical and psychological treatment compromised, there is a danger that he will not be respected as a person.

2.11 Psychiatric nursing

The nurse–patient relationship is in largely characterised by power — the patient being in the weaker position. The nurse's stronger position is derived to a great extent from special knowledge. This has many consequences for the patient in relation to labelling, and may involve more than simply giving the patient a bad name in such terms as 'difficult', 'rude' or 'demanding', which might be used by anyone.

Nurses, because of their special knowledge, are in a position to misuse as well as use legitimate clinical labels. Typical examples of this come from the field of psychiatry. A patient who is unsettled in his hospital surroundings may well display strange behaviour: he may be rather aggressive towards people, or emotionally very labile or he may refuse to talk to anyone. The words nurses use to describe this behaviour to one another may easily take on the apparently objective overtones of a clinical diagnosis. For example:

If a patient is rather low in spirits one evening because her husband is away on business and cannot visit her for a few days, the nurse might write in the Kardex, 'Feeling low tonight'. At the morning report she may say that the patient is 'a bit depressed'. The label 'depressed' then finds its way into the Kardex. The changeover of staff the next day means that the original user of the 'feeling low' term is no longer on duty, so that the reason — the husband's absence — gets lost and the 'depression' label gains momentum to the extent that the houseman is asked to prescribe something for the patient.

The dangers of using clinical labels which have quite specific meanings in psychiatry in this way are clear. Labelling of this kind is not in the best interests of either patients or nurses. If nurses are prepared to describe individual patients in derogatory or misleading terms, this is likely to affect the kind of care which they give. It also seems clear, from the literature on deviance, that persons are often labelled as deviant simply because they do not conform to the norm. But how do nurses decide what should be classed as normal? Even if a consensus about normality can be arrived at by nurses, what right does one group have to decide that the behaviour of another is not acceptable and thus refuse to tolerate it? The issue is not merely a clinical or social one, but one that has ethical implications relating to justice — in the sense of non-discrimination, and respect for persons — for example, the right to adequate care and treatment.

2.12 Minority groups

The hospital care of patients from minority religious or ethnic groups which have values or cultural practices differing from the majority of the population may well infringe their rights as individuals. In some cases, such as those of Jehovah's

Witnesses requiring blood transfusions, the moral issues can by very complex. An example is discussed in Chapter 4. But other cases may be resolvable if the nurses involved are reasonably sensitive and flexible. For example:

> A young nurse was in charge of a medical ward on night duty when a Jewish patient died. The nursing officer had warned her that she should move the patient from the ward before the relatives arrived, since once they started to mourn no one would be allowed to touch the body. In fact it was difficult to interfere in any way because the relatives had arrived and put candles round the bed some time before the patient died. The patient was moved into a side ward before he died — propped up on pillows and surrounded by his family. Later the nurse was reprimanded for not laying the body down flat in the normal way. But the nurse had realised that the Jewish faith insisted that no Gentile touch the patient and she had decided to abide by their rules.

The nurse's problem might have been solved in a practical way by ensuring that the family was on hand to carry out the funeral arrangements as they saw fit. The example does, however, illustrate problems which can and do arise when hospital policy or personnel are too rigid to accommodate the wishes of a minority group. The organisational machine — or mind — which insists that certain rules must be followed, can sometimes make it very difficult for a single nurse to do what he or she thinks is right for the patient. In the example given, for instance, a more junior nurse might have felt less secure in this position and, despite knowing about the Jewish faith, might have laid the patient flat. In circumstances of this kind, of course, as many more experienced nurses might well point out, the potential for flexibility within nursing and the individual nurse's capacity to work around the rules of the organisation may provide one way of resolving difficulties in protecting patients' rights. If, that is, a nurse knows why the hospital or health authority requires certain forms of behaviour from its nurses, she might then be in a position to bend the rules. For example, part of the routine surgical admission of patients includes the patient having a bath. Clearly, in some cases, depending on the patient's circumstances, this may be desirable if not indeed necessary. On the other hand to insist that every patient has a bath on admission not only may be unnecessary, but could give offence. It is not a particularly good way in which to build the relationship either. Thus, once nurses understand the reason for this traditional practice — namely, that at one time the general standard of hygiene was poor — they are in a position to attempt to waive the rules when appropriate. In justifying the desired action to seniors the nurse can invoke the reasoning behind the practice and demonstrate that as an inflexible rule it is not only redundant but also possibly counterproductive in terms of human relations. Such conduct on the part of a junior nurse may well require some courage. In nursing, as in life generally, there is never any ultimate guarantee that other people will accept what to us is simply listening to reason.

2.13 The nurse and dying patients

One of the most difficult aspects of nursing, and one which many nurses will admit they have never fully come to terms with, is the care of dying patients.

Lay and professional nursing of dying patients are obviously different experiences, not least by virtue of the ties of family or friendship which normally bind the dying to their lay carers. Even when death is a relief, the experiences of a lifetime's closeness, together with the memories of happiness and hurt have to be worked through; and especially when the inevitability of death is recognised, the working through may begin before death itself takes place. Professional nursing, by contrast, normally has no such fund of experiences to work upon. This does not mean that the professional nurse is not vulnerable to the hopes, fears and present experience of the dying individual. The experience of being in hospital is one which can allow people to speak more freely than normally about themselves; and the relationship between nurse and patient, however temporary, can be important to the patient, not least because of his dependence on the nursing staff. How important the relationship is to the nurse will depend, of course, on how far she heeds the advice not to become involved. Nurses, clearly, cannot build up close relationships with all of their patients, even when nursing is undertaken on a patient-centered rather than a task-oriented basis. Inevitably, for a great variety of reasons — perhaps because the patient reminds the nurse of a parent, perhaps because the patient chose this nurse for confiding domestic troubles to — some patients will be of particular importance to some nurses. Their encounter with one another, however brief, will leave unfinished business which nurses must work through in their own emotions.

As a professional, of course, the nurse will feel it important that her own emotional demands should not get in the way of skilled caring. This may be particularly difficult if the death of such a patient occurs when the nurse is feeling low for reasons rooted in her domestic or personal life. Under the circumstances, the pressure of other work may either give the nurse the strength to postpone working through emotions until she can find some time alone or it may be the final straw. Thus, the need to act in a professional way, given advantageous circumstances, may be what enables the nurse to get through this experience. On the other hand, the nurse's professional identity may itself complicate the pain of a patient's death — even where no particularly close nurse–patient relationship existed — by adding feelings of guilt and failure. The nurse's role, after all, is to sustain life and alleviate suffering. When it has not been possible to do either or both of these it is natural enough to ask why; and it is not unnatural, sometimes, to be less than rational about one's own possible errors or omissions.

The death of a patient may be difficult then because unfinished emotional business concerning a particular patient has to be worked through, or because anything less than a 'good' or timely death may create a sense of guilt and failure among professionals. The death of a patient may also be disturbing moreover when, for whatever reason, it brings home to those around a profound awareness of finality — that this is something no one can do anything whatever to alter. This knowledge, and with it the awareness of our own mortality and finite powers, is difficult for many of us to come to terms with, because one measure of our achievement as people is the capacity to live in the past and the future as well as the present. In the face of death, however, the past — much of which was preserved in the brain now dead — becomes much more tenuous, dependent now on the memories of others; while the present is empty, and the future — for the dead person at least — no longer exists. Some way of working through this experience, it is true, may be found by many people in religion, while for others the experience may provide the impetus to different kinds of action. But the realisation of finality and finitude, when a particular death evokes it, does need to be worked through in some way which provides a tolerable ard sustaining equilibrium between accepting this realisation and straining against it.

There are a variety of reasons, then, why the death of a particular patient may evoke strong feelings in a particular nurse, which may need to be addressed. Field (1984) gives some moving accounts of nurses' experiences with dying patients. If the deaths of all patients evoked such feelings, or if all nurses responded to one death in this way, professional nursing care of the patients, their relatives and other patients would not be possible. Yet, if nurses never gave expression to their feelings it would indicate that they were less than human rather than superhuman. The extent to which individual nurses do or do not allow themselves to express their feelings openly in such circumstances, may be a matter of professional judgement or personal moral choice.

Some degree of detachment from the situation has its positive aspects. Nurses have to continue to care for other patients when one patient has died. Allowing themselves to distance themselves from the death helps nurses to continue to function. It affords them some emotional protection and leaves them free to work according to the dictates of their professional knowledge rather than being entirely at the mercy of their own emotions. But sometimes tears are inevitable, and sometimes, when a whole ward has been aware of what has been happening behind the screens, it may be comforting to patients to know that nurses care enough to weep, provided that this does not cast doubts on their competence.

From the patients' point of view, evidence that the medical and nursing staff have 'failed' in another patient's case may be disturbing. For this reason it is understandable, when a patient has died in the night, that other patients, on asking where the patient is, may be told by a nurse that he has been moved to another part of the hospital. There are moral pressures on both sides of the argument here. If evasion is chosen, the case for not telling the whole truth cannot simply be taken for granted as being in the best interests of the patients, as the patronising attitudes of the past would have assumed, as it may be helpful to talk through with patients their fears about what has happened. Similarly, there may be good reasons for not giving information about a patient's death over the telephone to enquirers outside the immediate family, when there is doubt whether all the family have been informed, or whether they have had time to assimilate the knowledge. Related considerations also apply to summoning the family of a patient who may have died sooner than was expected. In subsequently breaking the news of a patient's death to his family, the way in which the truth is told is clearly as important as what is told.

When junior nurses ask how they should manage and what they should say and do when confronted with dying patients, the fact of death, and shocked relatives, they are often told: 'You will know what to say and do when it happens.' Clearly, the care of the dying and the bereaved is far more complex than this rather trite piece of advice would lead one to suppose. Glaser & Strauss (1965), discussed, among a number of other issues, the question of truth telling and openness with dying patients and their relatives, indicating the complexity of the issues involved.

Nowadays the first dying patient encountered by a first-year student may be the first dying person she has ever encountered, and even the experience of having to touch a dead human body may be something for which she is completely unprepared. Whether there are any adequate ways in which students can be prepared for such experiences is doubtful. There is in the end no substitute for the real thing. Nor is there any way of avoiding the feelings of pain, grief, guilt and helplessness which can be evoked in encounters with the dying, with death and with those who are left. Under these circumstances the moral pressure to put a brave face on things must usually, for practical reasons, be heeded. There are occasions however, when she cannot and perhaps should not, for the very good reason that some direct experience of her own human fallibility and frailty may be required to help the individual nurse recognise and accept the feelings of pain, grief, guilt and helplessness in the face of death. Without recognition and acceptance of feelings of this kind, they may lie buried and denied, so that in the future they either resurface in irrational and inappropriate ways which are difficult to control, or, if they are controlled, it can only be at the cost of deadening in the nurse those sensitivities which are essential for good nursing care.

In this chapter we have explored some of the moral conflicts involved in becoming and being a nurse. We have considered the conflicts between personal values and routine practice, in the transition from lay to professional status. We have looked also at the conflict between treating patients as people and not becoming involved, and discussed the dangers of labelling patients. These are, of course, only some of the moral issues which arise in patient care and the process of becoming and being a nurse. Perhaps they give some indication of the variety of moral choices which nurses have to make on a day to day basis, not only during their training but throughout their professional careers. In the next and subsequent chapters we shall examine a wide variety of other moral issues in nursing for the experienced and qualified nurse.

REFERENCES

Becker H S 1963 Outsiders: Studies in the sociology of deviance. Free Press of Glencoe, New York
Bond J, Bond S 1986 Sociology and health care: An introduction for nurses and other health care professionals. Churchill Livingstone, Edinburgh
Campbell A V 1985 Paid to care. SPCK, London
Emmet D 1966 Rules, roles and relations. Macmillan, London
Field D 1984 'We didn't want him to die on his own.' (Nurses' accounts of nursing dying patients). Journal of Advanced Nursing 9, 59–70
Freidson E 1970 Profession of medicine. Dodd Meads, New York, Chs 10–12
Glaser B G, Strauss A L 1965 Awareness of dying, Aldine, Chicago.
Henderson V 1966 The nature of nursing. Collier Macmillan, London
Lemert E M 1951 Social pathology. McGraw-Hill, New York.
Melia K M 1984 Student nurses' construction of occupational socialization. Sociology of Health and Illness 132–151
Melia K M 1987 Learning and working: The occupational socialisation of nurses, Tavistock, London
Parsons T 1970 The social system, Routledge & Kegan Paul, London, Ch 10
Ramsey P 1970 The patient as person. Yale University Press, New Haven, Conn.

3

Responsibility and accountability in nursing

Nurses form an occupational group which provides a wide variety of services within society. As such, nursing has organised itself into a bureaucratic style of working which places individual nurses within a formal structure. This structure determines, to a large extent, the behaviour of individual nurses; it puts limits on their range of activities; and it holds nurses accountable for their actions both as individuals and as members of the occupational group.

The organisational structure of nursing raises several issues which are pertinent to ethical debate about nursing. These issues can be divided into at least three areas: issues concerned with the nurse as a part of the nursing hierarchy; issues concerned with the nurse and other members of the health care team; and issues related to nurses' responsibility to their own profession. In order to understand many of the difficulties which nurses confront in their day-to-day work it may be helpful to begin by examining the hierarchical structure of nursing, and then to discuss the other two areas mentioned.

3.1 The nursing structure

The nursing service, unlike medicine, is organised according to the principles of line management. Essentially this means that qualified nurses, from the grade of staff nurse upwards, are organised into hierarchical grades within which each nurse is responsible for certain work and accountable to a senior nurse. Clearly, this is potentially a formalised system for 'buck-passing'. On the other hand, the system does not relieve the individual nurses of responsibility for their own actions. We will return to this point later.

Today's nursing organisation is, in general terms, a development of the Nightingale tradition which was established upon principles borrowed from military organisation; and something of the military tradition has obviously been retained in titles such as 'nursing officer'. The organisation for the delivery of nursing care instituted by Florence Nightingale was designed to allow for a wide range of ability within the service, and it worked as long as obedience of the military kind prevailed. As Carpenter (1977) put it: 'The beauty of this idea lay in its simplicity, serving in turn to unify the occupation into a single community stretching from the lowest ranking nurse to the highest ranking nurse. The crucial element in the situation was the power of the matron'.

This early band of nurse managers, matrons, by insisting upon obedience from their nurses, achieved a nursing service which would follow doctors' orders unquestioningly, yet which would not allow itself to be disciplined by doctors. The nursing service came under the direct control of the matrons. In the 1960s two administrative reorganisations replaced the matrons with a line management structure (Salmon 1966, Mayston 1969). This new structure resulted from the Salmon report's implicit call for an industrial model of professionalised management. Nursing was to be managed as might be any other workforce whose business it was to accomplish a task by means of group effort. The line management approach took the power held by the old-style matrons and shared it, to some extent, 'down the line' by giving different 'ranks' appropriate areas of responsibility and making them accountable for their work to an immediate superior. There have been some revisions of the original Salmon structure, but the line management principle still holds (Griffiths 1983).

This new bureaucratic model of operation poses problems for an occupational group which claims to be a profession. Autonomy and control over one's work are important hallmarks of a profession. Nursing has severe problems in this direction, not only because of the presence of the dominant profession of medicine, but also because the bureaucratic line management approach threatens to stifle professional judgement on the part of the individual nurse (Freidson 1970a, b). The medical profession gets around this difficulty by operating a collegial approach, which accepts each doctor as a professional who gives and seeks advice among colleagues and is open to judgement by his peers, but who is not held accountable for his day-to-day work to a management hierarchy. This difference in the organisational structures of medicine and nursing clearly presents problems when consultation and co-operation are required between individuals from the two professions.

As well as the military influence on nursing there was, of course, an even earlier religious influence. The older meaning of 'profession' has to do with the vows taken, or 'professed' by members of religious orders, some of whom were responsible for the care of the sick and poor in medieval hospitals, or hospices. These vows included obedience, also stressed in the military model, together with a strong sense of hierarchy. The religious model, too, emphasised the idea of the professed individual as a servant of others. This service emphasis was continued in Florence Nightingale's time. Nursing was not to be undertaken primarily for profit or financial gain. In practice, of course, nineteenth-century nursing seems to have been a means of providing work for the unmarriageable daughters of the middle and upper-middle classes. But the religious origins of its ideals also held out the promise of work which provided some measure of social worth. In this connection, the introduction of a capitalist rationality, which the Salmon report brought to the organisation of nursing, marks a further move away from its religious origins.

In the context of this discussion it is interesting to note how Florence Nightingale has been evoked in differing ways depending upon what image for nursing the author is trying to create. Whittaker & Olesen (1964) discussed the roles of Florence Nightingale — 'the lady with the lamp', 'the politician', 'the occupational status enhancer for nursing' — and the uses to which they are put.

The underlying rationale of the line management structure on which the Salmon and Mayston reorganisations were based provides a key to understanding the power and authority structures of nursing. Provision was made within the reorganisation for the inclusion of grades below that of the then nursing officer (number 7). Although the position in the line below charge nurse/ward sister has never been formalised, as it has above, the implicit hierarchical organisation from the most junior learner to the ward sister is obvious enough. In day-to-day practice on the wards the first-year learner will take an order from a second-year learner, as will the second-year learner from a third-year learner. From the first days of training, learners are made aware of the fact that they are the newest recruits; and as soon as another group arrives they immediately feel that they have moved a rung up the ladder. From these early days, therefore, a sense of the authority structure is acquired, even at the unofficial end of the hierarchy.

At this junior end of the line, line management principles are also recognised in other aspects of day-to-day practice. On any ward a senior nurse is recognised to be 'in charge'; during the daytime this nurse will almost certainly be qualified and is frequently the sister or charge nurse. With the shorter working week, however, the sister can only work five of the 14 daytime shifts; staff nurses and enrolled nurses will thus be 'in charge' for the remaining nine shifts. On night duty, however, a student nurse is likely to be left 'in charge' of a ward, with recourse to a night charge nurse who will be covering several wards. The remainder of the nurses on duty will take their work directives from the person who is in charge and will be accountable to that person for the work they are carrying out. Since there are a variety of ways in which the care of patients can be organised — in terms of 'who does what on this shift' — the nature of this organisation will have implications for the degree of responsibility and accountability of the individual nurse.

Crucial to the functioning of this hierarchical organisation is an understanding by all nurses of the routines and hospital ways of carrying out nursing and handling situations which arise in the course of nursing work. That is, nurses are made aware not only of their responsibilities in patient care, but also of the manner in which they should conduct themselves in the nursing hierarchy (Melia 1983). Within this routinised structure, individual nurses have to learn how to cope with their personal values and to make decisions about their actions as nurses.

3.2 Advantages and disadvantages of line management

The hierarchical system of line management has certain obvious advantages. One advantage is that it brings some power of decision-making closer to the area of patient care. A charge nurse or ward sister, for example, instead of having to ask the highest ranking nurse for extra help on a busy shift, might simply ask the immediate superior with whom they are in closer contact. On the other hand, requests involving greater changes may have to go to a higher authority, while policy decisions may come down the line to the ward sisters and charge nurses who have to put policy into practice whether or not they find it acceptable.

This form of management, then, puts nurses in a position where they are not always able to act in the way in which they as individuals might see fit. Depending upon the circumstances, this can be a positive or a negative feature of the hierarchical organisation of nursing. If, for example, the nurse involved is inexperienced or a learner, actions based on her own judgement might not be for the best. In such a case the hierarchical system and the restrictions it places upon the individual's behaviour may have advantages. For example:

A young patient decides that he is tired of waiting around the medical ward for the results of his tests and, despite his quite severe symptoms of a yet unknown cause, makes up his mind to take his own discharge. He waits until a quiet period in the afternoon when Sister has gone for her break and only junior nurses are in evidence on the ward. A junior nurse sees him dressing and he tells her he is leaving. He is very articulate, telling her that he fully understands his condition and has every right to leave. The junior nurse knows that she should tell a qualified member of staff, in the hope that they might be able to persuade the patient that it is in his own interest to stay. On the other hand, as an individual she can see his point: she feels moreover that he is a sensible young man who would get in touch with his general practitioner if he deteriorated in any way. Nevertheless, she follows the hospital-dictated procedure and, recognising that dealing with the situation falls outside her competence, she informs the staff nurse.

In this example, the advantage of the hierarchical organisation of nursing is that it affords protection to a less experienced member of staff. The junior nurse might well have
thought that there would be no harm in simply letting the
patient go — as indeed he had a legal as well as a moral right
so to do. However, as a nurse she was expected to follow
hospital policy, which dictated that she should inform a
senior nurse and that the patient must be required to sign
himself out in the presence of nurses, who in turn must sign
as witnesses of his discharge. In the event of the patient thus
leaving the hospital of his own will, the student would not
necessarily feel that she had compromised her own values,
or indeed the patient's, since he had achieved his end. What,
though, if he had been persuaded by senior staff to stay? The
student nurse might then have felt embarrassed at having let
him down by not following her own instincts. As an individual
she might have liked to see him go: at the very least she
might have wanted his interests as well as his rights
respected, and in the conflict between rights and interests
she might well have felt that it would be in his best interests
to stay. In this case the practical solution was arrived at in
terms of the student's position in the nursing hierarchy: she
passed responsibility 'up the line'. Having done so, however,
she still has to come to terms with the fact that had it not
been for her action the patient might well have got his own
way.

3.3 Conscientious objections

The above example illustrates some of the difficulties involved
when the nurse's personal view of the patient's best interests
conflicts with the official view which the nurse is expected to
follow. These difficulties are particularly acute if nurses feel
that they really must stand out against the official line, since
if they lose the support of colleagues they are placed in a
vulnerable position. In this connection the saying about there
being safety in numbers is particularly true when it comes to
making decisions about other people's lives.

There is, however, a further difficulty which may arise when
nurses decide to stand by their personal beliefs and perhaps
refuse to participate in certain kinds of treatment, or in a

particular treatment for one patient. This difficulty lies in the pressure the nurse's action places on those who do not exercise the right to abstain. One of the most obvious examples of this is the nurse's right not to participate in abortions. In the theatre this is a reasonably straightforward administrative problem, since only those nurses willing (or not objecting) to work with abortion lists will be employed there, although with a general theatre list this can still create difficulties for the staff who are left to cope after the conscientious objectors have absented themselves. The issue is becoming increasingly problematic for nurses when abortions are being carried out on the wards. The clauses of the 1967 Abortion Act do not allow for nurses refusing to participate in the pre- or post-operative care of a patient having an abortion. What, then, is the nurse's position in the care of a patient undergoing an induced abortion on the ward? Perhaps the nurse might reasonably refuse to have anything to do with the administration of the drug. But what should she do when the patient requires help when vomiting as a result of the abortion-inducing drugs? It seems unlikely that a nurse would refuse to help a patient in distress, but this does point up the limitations on the nurse's right to follow the dictates of conscience in this situation. One practical way out of such a problem might be to carry out ward-situated abortions only in areas where learners are not required to work; trained staff can choose where they will work. This solution, however, might open the way for a rather different kind of abortion service, not necessarily in the interests either of patients or of staff.

The underlying dilemma in the above discussion of the right of the nurse to opt out of abortion work is that if one nurse will not undertake certain work to which patients have a right, then another nurse must. A different aspect of this problem can be illustrated by a further example:

A man of 27 years with a wife and small daughter had hepatitis and renal failure. He had been on machine dialysis for three days a week. He was an in-patient, and although his progress was steady, it was not as good as expected. The consultant decided that the dialysis machine could be used to better effect for other patients. A decision was therefore made to take the patient off the machine and put him on diamorphine. This was done without much discussion and when the staff nurse was told to give the diamorphine injection she asked for time to discuss this with other staff. The nursing staff, except for the ward sister, decided to refuse to be involved with this injection because of the patient's age and his prognosis since coming off the dialysis machine and being given diamorphine. The night staff also refused. The night senior nurse, a third year student, was taken to the office and spoken to about her refusal, which upset her. Only the sister and the doctor gave the injection of diamorphine. The patient died before the next dialysis procedure was due.

This example illustrates the protection afforded by the hierarchy to the junior members of staff. However, it also demonstrates that even when the junior nursing staff are prepared to stand together, they cannot always expect support from their seniors. In this case, had the ward sister taken the view of the majority of the nurses, then the doctors would have had to take both prescriptive and practical responsibility for their treatment. As it was, the senior nurses further up the line of management made the third year student feel uncomfortable about the stance she took. This example raises considerations on both sides of the argument. If nurses are to decide on conscientious grounds how far they are prepared to go along with certain forms of treatment, the carrying-out of patient care might well become a much more difficult matter than at present. Nursing still works according to the Nightingale premise that nurses will do as they are told. But, as nurses become better informed, more vocal, more aware of their rights and more sensitive to the ethical implications of patient care, the nursing service may well need to look again at its terms and conditions of employment. A hard line which states that all care undertaken in a particular hospital will be undertaken by all nurses leaves the individual little scope for manoeuvre in moral matters. On the other hand, it would be administratively or operationally difficult to have a system of health care in which nurses could pick and choose among prescribed treatments.

Such issues were at stake in the case where a psychiatric nurse was dismissed for refusing to give a patient medication (Walsh 1982). This same nurse appealed against his dismissal and sought to take his case to the House of Lords, such was the seriousness of his disagreement with the medical treatment of a patient and his conviction that he and the junior nurses should have no part in it.

3.4 Knowledge and control in nurse management

Problems of a different kind again may be raised by the hier-archical structure of nursing when more junior members of staff have in fact more knowledge about a particular situation and are thus better suited to take relevant decisions. One example of this might be in an intensive care unit, where the sister in charge and her senior staff nurses may be in a better position than is the nursing officer to determine what staffing levels are required in the unit at any given time. The nursing officer may perhaps be out of touch with intensive care nursing, or may indeed never have had any clinical experi-ence in the area. Nursing officers are, nevertheless, in a position of authority which allows them to deploy staff in their units as they see fit. Even if this leaves the ward short-staffed, nurses are obliged to defer to the decisions of the senior staff.

At ward level also, the hierarchical order may require a junior nurse to obey the instructions of a less well-informed senior. Learner nurses encounter this problem when they come across a ward where the nursing care being carried out does not conform to the 'correct practice' they were taught in the college of nursing. A typical example of the problem is in the treatment of pressure areas. Some of the 'old school' approaches to preventive measures in skin care generally, and pressure areas in particular, have been shown to be not only ineffectual but possibly harmful.) The learner nurses face difficult situations when a ward sister asks them to carry out a procedure for a patient which the students know is not in the patient's best interest. The learner may well be able to cite the relevant research, to describe the preferred treatment and to justify the case. But the fact remains that as an unqualified junior questioning a senior, the position is awkward. The easiest practical solution to such a problem would probably be to follow the sister's wishes rather than pursue the matter with her tutor who might be more sympathetic to the view that nursing practice should be based on research findings. But what about the nurse's responsibility to the patient? There is also the question of litigation which, as in the United States, is becoming increasingly a matter for consideration in Britain. Patients are more aware of their rights as consumers in the NHS than has been the case in the past. Legal proceedings can be instigated if patients or relatives feel that they have a case against the medical or nursing staff with respect to their treatment and care. If learner nurses have reason to believe that the care they are being asked to give by seniors could be harmful to the patients, then a confrontation with the senior nurse might seem the only course open to them. Such behaviour might not be consistent with the line of authority approach, but it might be morally and legally prudent in such a case.

3.5 Responsibility, ward organisation and record-keeping

As has already been mentioned, the style of organisation on a ward can have implications for the amount of responsibility an individual nurse carries. We can distinguish two main styles of ward organisation: one, commonly referred to as patient allocation, where the patient is the central focus; and one where tasks and routine are the main features. Patient allocation means that each nurse is assigned one or more patients and is responsible for their care. The use of detailed care plans, in which individualised instructions for the patient's care can be found, is a characteristic of this style of ward management. These care plans may also be used for the other style of organisation, however, where they can be combined and translated into routine tasks in terms of the whole ward. In a patient allocation system, the individual nurse is responsible for all the care of one or more patients. In many ways this puts more pressure on the nurse than if she were simply part of the ward work force with a share in the care of all patients. If nurses know that they are responsible simply for, say, fluids and fluid balance charts for the whole ward, then they can go about the day's tasks in a fairly routine way without taking responsibility for any single patient: while one nurse takes care of fluids, others in turn will attend to baths, dressings, recording and so forth for the same patients. Thus the patients, or at least their needs, are fragmented and distributed among the nurses, who have collective responsibility for the care: but the weight of responsibility falls upon the nurses in charge who allocated the tasks.

One of the common arguments against patient allocation is that more staff are required to put it into practice. But in a study of student nurses' views on nursing (Melia 1981) a number of students recorded a positive preference for routine and a task-centred approach because it represented a foolproof system for getting through the work without items of care being missed out. On these grounds it can be argued that the certainty which a routine provides can benefit the patients, who may rest assured that their basic needs will be met. Junior nurses also may gain security by avoiding the stress of being wholly responsible for any one patient. Against this view, however, must be set the possible therapeutic benefits of a patient-centred approach and its advantages in terms of work satisfaction for many nurses.

Whichever style of organisation is adopted, however, responsibility ultimately falls on one member or other of the nursing staff, whether it be the nurse wholly responsible for a particular patient or the nurse in charge of a task-oriented ward. In practice, of course, the nurse's employer, the health authority, is also vicariously responsible for her actions or omissions, and while individual nurses may be sued by patients or relatives along with the health authority, it is recognised that the latter is most likely to be able to pay any damages awarded by the court. On the other hand, it is worth noting that the employing authority is then entitled to try to recover its costs from the individual nurse. In such circumstances, record-keeping is clearly a crucial factor. How the patient has been treated can be seen from accurate notes kept and signed by the nurses involved in the case; then, should there be any dispute, a statement of the facts is available. The kind of issues involved can be illustrated by an example:

An elderly patient, who was unable to walk, persisted in getting out of bed, unaided, during the night and repeatedly fell to the floor. Because of the layout of the ward and the lack of staff, constant observation was not possible. Cot-sides were not used in the unit and extra sedation was not recommended. The accident forms often amounted to three a night, although not every night. The senior nursing officer questioned the number of forms and recommended that it was not necessary to fill these in at each incident, because of the frequency with which these falls occurred.

The nurse who had been filling in the forms then had to ask herself whether she should continue to do so, to cover herself from the legal aspect, or whether she should carry out her senior's instructions.

In this case the records concerned — the hospital accident forms — were additional to the nursing care records. The senior nurse manager looked at the situation in terms of wasted time and effort: but the nurse who was most immediately involved was anxious to follow the hospital procedure, not least for her own protection.

The matter of record-keeping was raised in cases where parents complained about lack of information received from health visitors in connection with immunisation. The question of whether a health visitor could be sued for omitting to make parents aware of all the side effects and possible dangers associated with vaccination has also arisen. Obviously, health visitors do not record every word of their conversation with clients, so that in court it could well be the client's word against the health visitor's. A history of clear and full record-keeping would be in the health visitor's interest if a case were to be brought. Aside from the legal issue, and it has to be said that individual health visitors are far less likely to be sued than their health authorities, there is a more basic moral point. For health visitors a prime professional responsibility is preventive health care. When they encounter individual parents who want to know what they think as individuals about vaccination, when asked for instance, 'What if it were your child?', the health visitor has to balance her own personal concern for that particular family with her wider remit of achieving widespread immunity in the population (Whincup 1982).

3.6 The nurse and the health care team

In the context of the health care team, possibly the greatest scope for conflict is in the relationship between nursing and medical practice. Just as there is a power dimension to the relationship between patient and nurse so there is in the relationship between nurse and doctor. The source of the medical profession's authority and power lies in the fact that doctors carry legal responsibility for decisions about patient care and treatment. As we have seen in the cases of conscientious objection, discussed earlier, conflict or disagreements between nurses and doctors arise over who has ultimate authority and control over patient care. Nurses may be left with responsibility for patients, yet have no authority to change doctors' orders nor legal right to refuse to carry out medical instructions even if they object.

There are two factors related to the structure of medicine and nursing which are potential sources of conflict. The first factor, already mentioned, is the difference between the collegial organisation of medicine and the hierarchical organisation of nursing. The collegial mode is based upon professional trust, individual discretion and an informal system of regulation by one's peers: in practice, a junior doctor will seek advice from and be guided by his more experienced senior colleagues, but with much less need for a formal line of command than in nursing. At the ward level, this can create problems. If, for example, a registrar acts in some way which contravenes hospital policy, he enjoys greater freedom to do so than does the ward sister who is associated with this action. The registrar may, say, leave the ward and ask to be telephoned if a seriously ill patient's condition deteriorates. He may then find it perfectly acceptable to prescribe medication over the telephone, await the outcome and decide to return only if certain changes occur. This action may meet the approval of his colleagues, and the ward sister, as an individual, may consider it perfectly reasonable, not least because the patient will benefit from receiving the drug sooner than if he had to wait for the doctor's return. However, the ward sisters and charge nurses will also be aware that to order drugs over the telephone is against the hospital policy which they are supposed to implement, and that if they comply with the registrar's wishes they will not enjoy the support of their seniors. This is only one example of the kinds of conflict which arise when these two front-line professionals try to work together. At a day-to-day level both must be able to co-operate in planning the care of the patients: the smooth and efficient running of the ward depends on the working relationship between doctor and nurse at this level. The nursing staff, however, are to some extent bound by the rules involved in being the hospital's 'clinical civil service', and this can bring them into conflict with doctors who have more of the status of free agents who practise their craft in hospitals.

The second potential source of conflict in the nurse–doctor relationship lies in the nature of nursing as an occupation. Nursing can be said to be in part dependent upon and in part independent of medical practice. There are, clearly, some areas of nursing work which mostly have to do with carrying out the care prescribed by doctors. In this sense the nurse is simply following orders. There are, however, other areas of care, mostly to do with the patient's comfort and social well-being, in which the nurse should take action independent of medicine. Doctors have a tendency to see nursing as an entirely dependent profession, which exists to help them. Some nurses are happy to go along with this working definition. Others prefer to develop their nursing skills, arrive at decisions on how best they think the patient might be cared for, and form what could be called a nursing opinion. Having formed an opinion, the nurse might then wish to question the work of the doctor; at a level more pragmatic than ethical, the nurse might, for example, question the wisdom of his prescription. Often an experienced ward sister will be in a position to advise a more junior doctor upon the best treatment in cases of which she has had past experience. If the doctor is not prepared to listen to her opinion or, having listened, ignores it, the nurse is then faced with the choice between letting the matter drop, possibly to the detriment of the patient on the grounds that 'the doctor knows best', or pressing her opinion to the extent of calling in a senior doctor or refusing to co-operate in the treatment. On the military analogy, the sister may then marshal troops and dictate to nursing staff what the nursing strategy will be. In the case of such confrontation, teamwork breaks down and the issue moves from the pragmatic area to the ethical. The determining factor in the outcome of such conflicts often lies in the answer to the question about who is ultimately responsible. Nurses, to their own satisfaction, might have a right to a nursing opinion and also a right to challenge medical staff. But what of the responsibility? The 'contract' which the patient enters into when he is ill is between patient and doctor. The patient is ultimately the doctor's responsibility.

Difficulties of this kind are often most acute in areas such as geriatric medicine, terminal care, psychiatry and obstetrics where team decisions are often taken but where the responsibility is ultimately that of the doctor. Because of this, the teamwork ideal may be difficult to translate into practice. Further difficulties can be caused by the fact that health care professions and occupations other than medicine and nursing may each have their own hierarchies, lines of accountability, rules, regulations and working practices. Many decisions that directly affect the care of patients and the running of wards — from cleaning to hospital meals, portering to the ambulance service — are outside the control of the sister and her ward staff, however much patients and their relatives may imagine that they are responsible.

Nurses are largely responsible for seeing that patients get the care that they require. Judgements about how to spread nursing time among a group of patients have to be made; these are in part clinical and in part moral judgements, they are usually described as professional judgements. Nurses are exhorted in a generalised and often emotional sense to care for patients, at the same time they have to make decisions about how and where to distribute their time and care. A professional nursing service must make fair decisions on the basis of nursing knowledge, not on some generalised emotive ethic of 'caring'. Professional nursing, if it is to distinguish itself from lay nursing, must operate according to some notion of justice based on nursing expertise when it comes to determining how much time and care can be devoted to individual patients. The only real justification for having trained nurses (an expensive commodity) is the fact that they have specialist knowledge and skills upon which to base their work as opposed to the altruism that guides lay carers. This expertise allows professional nurses to meet the demands made by justice. To treat a ward full of patients justly requires knowledge and skill and an ability to make appropriate judgements on the basis of that knowledge. Justice does not have to do with an *equal* distribution of time and care among all patients; rather, it demands that sensible decisions are made about the *equitable* allocation of nursing time and effort relative to objectively assessed need. If, for example, there is a violent patient causing disruption on a ward, it is in the best interests of all patients that nurses concentrate their efforts on that patient until such time as he has been calmed. This might mean that a meal is served late, or a routine drug round is delayed. Even though the majority of patients received no attention for a period of time, and indeed had their meals and medication delayed, while the patient took up the total nurse attention available, the nurses can be said to have acted in the best interests of all the patients. Professional nursing decisions, then, are made on the basis of an appeal to justice rather than to a more simplistic ethic of caring.

3.7 Responsibility to the profession

Professional groups which enjoy a monopoly in determining the service they provide must also accept responsibility for their standards of practice. Nurses, as a professional group, are clearly concerned about standards of care.

One has only to look at the nursing press or reports from nursing conferences to see that a preoccupation with standards and the quality of patient care is one which many nurses share. Typically, the professions claim to have knowledge and skills which allow their members to give some form of service. The fact that the service is of a specialised nature with a theoretical base makes it difficult for a lay person to judge the performance of professionals. For this reason, the professions themselves seek to develop ways of assuring society that it will be protected from any undesirable consequences of the professional monopoly. To this end, the profession sets its own standards of practice, trains its own recruits, disciplines its members and strives to maintain its standards. The arguments for this practice centre on the fact that a specialist knowledge is required in order to understand professional behaviour, and so self-regulation is the most effective way to maintain standards. The difficulty, however, is that the closed nature of the professional organisation prevents any independent viewpoint being brought to bear on the profession's practice.

The fact that professionals are not above the law goes some way to alleviating any fears which society might have about abuse of privileged positions. The courts provide a means of regulating the conduct of professionals whose conduct moves

outside the law. While the law may not be the most appropriate medium for resolving ethical issues, it does have the
virtue of impartiality and can set limits to the harmful potential of monopoly power. On the other hand, while it would
be undesirable to have a medical profession whose members
were never required to justify their actions, the complexities
of medical decision-making are such that a legalistic approach
to a debate about its rights and wrongs may be unhelpful. For
example:

A nurse as part of an intensive care team has been involved in the
care of a brain-damaged patient. After the patient has been on a
respirator for a few days, the physicians establish that brain death
has occurred. After discussion with the relatives and the nursing
staff, the doctor in charge of the patient's case decides that the
respirator should be turned off and the patient's heart left to stop.
The whole team is in complete agreement with the decision and the
nurse who has been looking after the patient turns off the machine.

If, in such a case, circumstances for some reason lead to
a court hearing because the life support machine has been
switched off, the complex series of events which led up to
switching off the machine might sound very different in a
court room. The way in which evidence is handled often
leaves little scope for an explanation of all the surrounding
circumstances. Thus the description of events might be interpreted by a lay jury in a way very different from that of
informed medical and nursing opinion. On the other hand
again, is it not right that an outside view should be sought?
Will a professional group not simply confirm its own conduct
and because of familiarity fail to see the flaws in its practice
which a lay person might see? Doubts of this kind cannot be
dismissed out of hand, not least because even when cases
come to the courts the profession's own definition of events
is influential. As McCall Smith remarked in his discussion of
the legal aspects of the RCN Code (Journal of Medical Ethics
1977), 'The law may ultimately be called upon to define what
is acceptable practice on the part of the professions but it
tends to do so on the basis of what the professions themselves suggest. The law, then, looks for guidance to
professional consensus, while the professions naturally look
to the law for a statement of what they can or cannot do.' In
the light of this circular relationship between consensus and

the law, McCall Smith concludes, 'The promulgation of a code of professional conduct is of major legal significance, in that it can be influential in the moulding of legal attitudes.'

The judge's summing up in the case of the late Dr Leonard Arthur accused of murdering a Down's syndrome baby, underscored the point (Brahams & Brahams 1983). After hearing expert medical opinion on the treatment of severely handicapped neonates, the judge said, 'Whatever ethics a profession might evolve they could not stand on their own or survive if they were in conflict with the law. . . . I imagine you will think long and hard before concluding that doctors of the eminence we have here have evolved standards that amount to committing a crime.'

From the profession's point of view, also, codes of ethics or codes of conduct are important — both as ways of proclaiming publicly their trustworthiness and as a means of giving their members some guidance as to their practice. In this connection it is perhaps useful to think of a profession's standards on the one hand at a micro-level, in the sense of how individual members behave towards their patients, clients and colleagues, and on the other hand at a macro-level where the professional ethic can be seen as something the whole profession upholds and which can be invoked by individual members to support their behaviour. In discussing codes of ethics in nursing, we will be concerned with both levels at which codes operate.

3.8 Codes of ethics

There are several codes of ethics to which we might turn in order to gain some idea of their form and purpose (UKCC 1983). Until this century, the medical profession in Britain has never had an agreed code of ethics, although the highly regarded, if rarely read, Hippocratic Oath serves as an 'ethical flag'. Since World War II the British Medical Association has taken a prominent role in the World Medical Association and is a signatory to the International Code of Medical Ethics and various Declarations of the World Medical Association (see Dictionary of Medical Ethics). The American Medical Association (AMA 1977), however, followed what it saw as a British lead when in 1848 it adopted a code of ethics based on an earlier code drawn up by the Manchester physician, Thomas Percival in 1849 (Parker 1977).

The established professions tend to make explicit the moral standards which guide their professional conduct and then rely on the integrity of their members to carry out their work in the clients' best interests (British Medical Association 1984). Wilding (1982) has described codes of ethics and conduct as 'campaign documents prepared in a search for privilege and power, or in their justification.' Few would go so far, but it has to be said that the practice of producing ethical codes is probably linked with the desire of certain occupations to claim professional status.

Today British doctors accept the Hippocratic Oath in its more up-to-date formulation, namely the International Code of Medical Ethics as providing general guidelines for medical practice (Veatch 1977). In recent times written codes and declarations in medicine have sought to prevent the decline of medical standards. Alternatively, they may be written as a response to some particular ethical debate. The 1947 Nuremberg Code, concerned with permissible medical experiments, for example, was drawn up after revelations about Nazi war crimes involving medical experiments on human subjects. Further examples of codes drawn up by the World Medical Association include: the Declaration of Helsinki (1964 and 1975) on research involving human subjects; the Declaration of Sydney (1968), on the determination of the time of death; the Declaration of Oslo (1970), on therapeutic abortion; and the Declaration of Tokyo (1975), on torture, degrading treatment and punishment. Ethical guidelines for psychiatrists were drawn up by the World Psychiatric Association in the Declaration of Hawaii (1977) (Duncan et al 1981).

Nursing and social work are two major caring professions which have followed the example of medicine and produced their own codes of ethics. Again, we have to look to America to find one of the earliest codes. In 1893, at the Farrand Training School for Nurses at the Harper Hospital of Detroit, Lystra Grecter, principal of the school, devised the Nightingale Pledge (Robinson 1946). By this pledge, graduates of the school promised, '[to] pass my life in purity and to practise my profession faithfully. I will abstain from whatever is deleterious and mischievous and will not take or administer any harmful drug.' There was no connection between this pledge and Florence Nightingale; it would appear, however, that Lystra Grecter felt that the name of Nightingale would add weight to the pledge.

It was some time before the ethical codes in nursing, with which we are familiar today, were developed. In 1950 the American Nurses Association produced its Code for Nurses. The early versions of the code were mainly prescriptive, Tait said: 'Identifying codes of both personal and professional behaviour, describing appropriate relationships with physicians and other health care professionals.' But the latest code, 'while remaining prescriptive, depends more upon the nurse's accountability to the client' (Tait 1977). Along with the code there are 'interpretive statements', which render the code more than a list of do's and dont's. The Royal College of Nursing adopted this approach in 1976 when it drew up its code of Professional Conduct (RCN 1976). The International Council of Nurses first produced its Code of Ethics in 1953; this was revised in 1965 and replaced in 1973, when the Council adopted the Code for Nurses: Ethical Concepts Applied to Nursing (ICN 1973).

The latest professional code for nurses in Britain is the UK Central Council's Code of professional Conduct (UKCC 1983). This code was drawn up following the Nurses, Midwives and Health Visitors Act 1979, which gave the UKCC powers including, 'That of giving advice in such a manner as it thinks fit on standards of professional conduct.' The authors of this code could be said to have taken a rather narrow view of a professional code in so far as it can be seen in large part to be a checklist against which alleged cases of professional misconduct might be judged. In many ways the opening remarks in this code could have stood in its stead. The more detailed clauses which follow tend to undermine the professional idealism proclaimed at the outset.

If nurses are to work as members of multidisciplinary teams, it is perhaps relevant here to take a brief look at the social worker's approach to the question of professional ethics. The American National Association of Social Workers formulated its ethical code in 1960 (Morris et al 1971), but it was not until 1976 that the British Association of Social Workers adopted its code (BASW 1977). Clark & Asquith

(1985) remarked: 'If the generations of American and British social workers who practised before these dates managed well enough without a formalised code of ethics, it is at least questionable that a formal statement adds anything to their inheritor's understanding. Whatever the improvements in knowledge that may have been attained by later generations, it is not suggested that the first social workers were less ethical than modern ones.' Clark & Asquith went on to say, as it has already been argued in the case of nursing, that the move towards a production of codes goes hand in hand with aspirations for professional status. They discussed the BASW Code and its similarities with the ICN Code for Nurses. They concluded that since much that is contained in these codes is descriptive rather than prescriptive, 'It is unclear in what sense these can be ethical statements . . . the principles purportedly underlying the codes are not translated into any clear or complete statement of rights and duties, indeed the social work codes seem to have more to say about professionals' rights than clients'.'

What, then, are the limitations of ethical codes? Let us, by way of illustration, examine just one part of the Declaration of Oslo, on therapeutic abortion, which states (Clause 6): 'If a doctor considers that his convictions do not allow him to advise or perform an abortion, he may withdraw while ensuring the continuity of [medical] care by a qualified colleague.'

At first sight this clause appears to provide a fairly straight-forward guideline which the doctor might follow. This kind of conscience clause allows the doctor the right of consci-entious objection, that is, to refuse to perform any procedure which is against his principles. It does, however, leave the potential for practical difficulties. If no colleague is available to provide the care (either, say, in a routine case or if his colleagues are equally opposed to abortion), can the indi-vidual doctor demand the right to work according to his beliefs if these are at variance with those of many of his patients?

In practice, then, codes of ethics clearly have their limi-tations and cannot be seen as always providing the answer to day-to-day moral dilemmas. What such codes can do, however, is to set out the general rights, duties, values and policies which should govern professional practice. As such, they provide a means of laying down standards of conduct which a profession might expect its members to meet. Indeed, this is recognised in the RCN (1976) discussion document. The introduction states: 'No code can do justice to every individual case and therefore any set of principles must remain constantly open to discussion both within the nursing profession and outside it.' The same document supplies a further reason for having an ethical code: 'To provide a clear and comprehensive document for further discussion, particularly during training.'

The code thus states the ideal professional standards in a clear way which can be recognised as a description of the desired behaviour of professionals. If, as an individual, a nurse is unsure of the position that she should adopt in some situation, the code can supply some guidance. For example, if nurses are unhappy about a particular treatment which a dying patient is receiving, they might feel that as individuals they have no option other than to follow the doctor's instructions.

However, not only do nurses have the right but it is also their duty to express an opinion about the effect of treatment on patients. While nurses might feel diffident about making an opinion known, especially if they are expressing views which run counter to those of the doctor who is prescribing the care, they can find support for their action in the code of ethics. The RCN Code for example, states: 'Measures which jeopardise the safety of patients, such as unnecessary treatment, hazardous experimental procedures and the withdrawal of professional services during employment disputes should be actively opposed by the profession as a whole.' Individual nurses must live up to this code and express opinions when they have them. Nurses can be said to have a duty to the profession to behave in such a way, even though the organisation within which they work historically gives more weight to doctors' opinions.

3.9 Responsibility for professional standards

If nurses are to be accountable for their care in a professional sense they also have a duty to keep up to date in the knowledge base of their profession. It is not sufficient that a nurse pass her final examinations, qualify and then never consider it necessary to continue her education. Nurses must be responsible for the care they give, and it cannot be claimed that because nurses work according to doctors' orders they are exempt from any responsibility. For example, if a nurse thinks that a doctor's prescription contains the wrong dose of the drug, she has a duty to question it, and if there is still doubt, to refuse to give the drug. Nurses, along with the doctor, might be charged with negligence, if they failed to recognise the incorrectly prescribed dosage of a commonly known drug such as digoxin.

One might, of course, argue that it is the doctor's business to get the prescriptions right and that the nurse cannot be held responsible. However, nurses take responsibility for their actions and must carry out patient care in an intelligent way which includes recognising potential harm to her patients. Again, from a code of ethics, this time from the ICN (1973): 'The nurse takes appropriate action to safeguard the individual when his care is endangered by a co-worker or any other person.' The general point about responsibility for professional standards is also made by the RCN Code (1976): 'The professional authority of nurses is based upon their training and experience in day-to-day care of ill persons at home or in hospital; and the enhancement of positive health in the community at large. All members of the nursing profession have a responsibility to continue to develop their knowledge and skill in these matters.'

In order to maintain professional standards, then, nurses must inform themselves of advances in knowledge of nursing care. Not only must the profession ensure that its new recruits achieve a certain standard before they are allowed to practise; but it must also make certain that its established members maintain those standards. Indeed, because nurse training involves a substantial amount of learning on the job, it is imperative that practitioners keep themselves up to date so that the learners are exposed to practice of the right standard.

Practice based on sound principles and established empirical evidence might distinguish a professional from a lay approach to activity in a given field. At a macro-level the profession must ensure that its standards of practice are supported by a sound theoretical base. At a more individual or micro-level, the practitioners must be sure their practice is up to date.

In the case of nursing, much of the work which nurses undertake was for a long time, and in some instances still is, based upon tradition rather than research. However, for some years now nursing research has been undertaken and its findings made available to the profession. This means that the individual nurse can no longer plead ignorance if she chooses to follow tradition rather than a proven form of treatment. A good example of this, which we have already mentioned, is the care of pressure areas and the treatment of pressure sores. Even after publication of condemnatory findings (Norton 1975) nurses continued to rub soap and water, spirit and a variety of other dubious applications on patients' skin. For learner nurses this particular example might pose ethical difficulties. From the college of nursing students will have been supplied with the latest research-based information in relation to the care of pressure areas; yet on the ward they could be told that the sister's policy involves a treatment which the student knows has been shown to be harmful. Given that nurses are supposed to be not only responsible for their actions but also morally accountable for them, this student's choice between following the teachings of the college and obeying the ward sister is a difficult one. In this particular example, because of the workings of the nursing hierarchy, it might also be hard for the student to invoke the professional code of practice in defence of disregarding the sister's instructions (RCN 1976).

Clearly the professional macro-level and the individual micro-level converge at some point and share responsibility for advancing the knowledge of the discipline. Accurate and meaningful record-keeping on the part of the nurse can provide the data required to evaluate present practice. Thus, while each individual nurse will not be a researcher as such, she should take a responsible attitude towards her nursing record-keeping in order that the effects of X upon Y in nursing care can be documented. The nursing process is an attempt at such an approach to nursing. For example, toilet practices with elderly incontinent patients could be recorded carefully, and after a period the success of individual programmes could be assessed in terms of the degree of continence attained. Nurses might take a lead from their medical colleagues in this respect. Doctors do not all follow identical treatment patterns with patients with similar conditions. For instance, coronary care might vary from one doctor to the next with equally successful results. It matters little that the treatments are different; what does matter is that doctors take note of the effects of their treatment and thus build up a working repertoire of medical practice, based, of course, upon the theory available to all those practising medicine but refined according to their observations. Furthermore, if a doctor arrives at a particularly successful way of treating a condition he will communicate this to his colleagues through the professional journals.

3.10 Reporting on colleagues

Aside from having a personal individual responsibility for their own practice and maintenance of professional standards, nurses also have a wider responsibility to the nursing profession. This means that they should be prepared to report poor standards of care and nursing which is not practised in accordance with the professional standard, when they encounter it. This presents perhaps the most trying moral difficulties of all.

If poor practice is to be curbed it must be reported and it is a fact of life that often the person best placed to observe and report bad practice on the part of a nurse will be another nurse. What price professional loyalty then? If a nurse sees one of her colleagues maltreating a patient, for example an elderly patient or a mentally handicapped person, what is she to do? The nurse's own private morality will dictate that the action was wrong and that the correct line of action would be to report the incident. Still at an individual level, the nurse might feel something of a 'sneak' telling tales about another individual's action. Yet nurses are likely to be able to ignore these feelings because of the rights of the maltreated patient whose position they are really defending. Nurses then have the profession to contend with. The colleague has brought disgrace upon the profession to which she belongs. Nurses are trusted by patients, indeed by society as a whole, to be caring and kind. They are put in a position of trust by virtue of having the care and, in many senses, the charge of the lives of other individuals. The nurse who witnesses a colleague's malpractice is then faced with a choice between exposing the colleague and risking publicity (and the damage to the professional image which goes with it), and keeping quiet, hence betraying the patient's trust.

If the nurse faced with this choice is a learner then the dilemma is more acute. Aside from the conflict for her between the profession and the trust of patients, she has her own future career as a nurse to consider. Beardshaw (1981) asked: 'Are nurses able to protect their patients' interests by speaking up when they are abused?' Often they are not. They may be forced to stand by when individual patients are ill-treated or when poor conditions deprive them of adequate care. Their silence is enforced by feelings of impotence and by fears of reprisals. The victimisation of some nurses who have spoken up about abuse is a vivid illustration that these fears can be well founded.

If a nurse complains about the conduct of another nurse, then she has to consider whether she will be listened to, be believed, what it will do to her other relationships within the hospital and ultimately to her career prospects. Even though it might be a patient's suffering which is at stake, it is a difficult thing to 'blow the whistle' on one's colleagues, as Beardshaw puts it. One DNE's comment sums it up: 'Students still comment as follows: "We would be told off for inter-fering"; "No one would take any notice of me"; "I need a job in the future". All worry about victimisation' (Beardshaw 1981).

Beardshaw (1981) pointed out the difficulties for student nurses which exist in the ICN Code for Nurses. How can the nurse follow the ICN Code and take appropriate action to safeguard the individual when his care is endangered by a co-worker or any other person, when the nurse is subject to both the medical profession and the nursing hierarchy? The position of the student nurse, she concluded, 'Encapsulates an essential contradiction of nursing professionalism — a professional waiting for orders — where emphasis on obedience to authority dilutes the professional responsibility of individual nurses.'

In this chapter we have looked at some of the ethical issues which arise out of working in a hierarchy, working as a member of a health care team and from having a responsibility to a professional group. Some time has been spent considering codes of ethics and their utility. It is clear that the issues are so wide-ranging and complex that no code can be more than a guide to professional conduct. It can, to borrow the words of Florence Nightingale, do the profession no harm to have an ethical code, for in the code lie the means of safeguarding the public and a reminder to the profession of the need to maintain standards. Codes of ethics will, however, never provide a panacea. It is the prevailing moral climate within the profession which will exert the most influence at the end of the day. Nurses, along with their colleagues in the caring professions, must develop a sense of moral judgement in their work and recognise that health care work is a moral enterprise.

REFERENCES

American Nurses Association 1977 Code for nurses (1950, revised 1976) Reproduced and discussed in: Tait B L 1977 The nurse's dilemma: Ethical considerations in nursing practice. ICN, Geneva, pp 77–93
Beardshaw V 1981 Conscientious objectors at work. Social Audit, London p 2
Brahams D, Brahams M 1983 The Arthur case — a proposal for legislation. Journal of Medical Ethics 9, 12–15
British Association of Social Workers (BASW) 1977 The social work task. BASW, Birmingham
British Medical Association 1984 Handbook of medical ethics. BMA, London. (A somewhat discursive document — covering aspects of medical etiquette and 'ethics')
Carpenter M 1977 The new managerialism and professionalism in nursing. In: Stacey M et al Health and the division of labour. Croom Helm, London
Clark C L, Asquith S 1985 Social work and social philosophy: A guide for practice. Routledge & Kegan Paul, London, p 84
Duncan A S, Dunstan G R, Welbourn R B 1981 Dictionary of medical ethics, revised edn. Darton, Longman & Todd, London. (See Declarations of the World Medical Association)
Freidson E 1970a Profession of medicine. Dodd Mead, New York
Freidson E 1970b Professional dominance. Dodd Mead, New York
Griffiths R 1983 NHS management inquiry. (Letter to Secretary of State) London

International Council of Nurses 1973 Code for Nurses: Ethical Concepts applied to nursing. ICN, Geneva. (This code was adopted in May 1973 in Mexico. It replaces the ICN Code of Ethics, adopted in Sao Paolo, Brazil, in 1953 and revised in 1965. See International Nursing Review Vol 20, No.25, 1973)

Journal of Medical Ethics 1977 Royal College of Nursing Code of Professional Conduct (discussion). Journal of Medical Ethics 3(3), 122

Mayston 1969 Report of the working party on management structure of the local authority nursing services (Mayston Report). HMSO, London

Melia K M 1981 Student nurses' accounts of their work and training: A qualitative analysis. Unpublished PhD thesis, University of Edinburgh

Melia K M 1983 1. Students' views of nursing, 2. Just passing through. Nursing Times. May 18, 26–27

Morris R et al (eds) 1971 Profession of social work: Code of Ethics. In: Encyclopaedia of social work (16th issue). National Association of Social Workers, New York

Norton D 1975 Research and the problem of pressure sores. Nursing Times 140, 65–67

Parker J H 1977 Of professional conduct. Reprinted from Thomas Percival, Medical ethics, 3rd edn, Oxford, 1849, pp 27–68. In: Reiser S J, Dyck A, Curran W J Ethics in Medicine. MIT Press, Cambridge, Mass., pp 18–25

Reiser S J, Dyck A, Curran W J 1977 Ethics in medicine: Historical perspectives and contemporary concerns. MIT Press, Cambridge, Mass., pp 26–34

Robinson V 1946 White Caps. Lippincott, New York

Royal College of Nursing 1976 Code of Professional Conduct: A discussion document, RCN, London. (Reproduced in JME 1977 3(3))

Salmon 1966 Report of the committee on senior nursing staff structure. (Salmon Report): HMSO, London

Tait B L 1977 (See American Nurses Association 1977 above)

UKCC 1983/84 The Code of Professional Conduct for the Nurse, Midwife and Health Visitor, United Kingdom Central Council for Nursing, Midwifery and Health Visiting, London

Veatch R M 1977 Case studies in medical ethics. Harvard University Press, London, pp 351–356. (This code was adopted by the Third General Assembly of the World Medical Association in London in 1949. It followed acceptance of the Declaration of Geneva, made at the General Assembly of the WMA in Geneva in 1948 (amended in 1986). Both Declaration and Code are reproduced in Veatch)

Walsh P 1982 Why I am opposing the doctors. (Interview by Cherrill Hicks.) Nursing Times Sept 22, 1579–1580

Whincup M 1982 The duties of a health visitor. Nursing Times 77 (13), 567–568. (Legal issues are often intrinsically bound up with ethical ones. Two useful references in this area are: Young A P 1981 Legal problems in nursing practice. Harper & Row, London. Pyne R H 1981 Professional discipline in nursing — theory and practice. Blackwell, Oxford)

Whittaker E, Olesen V 1964 The faces of Florence Nightingale: functions of the heroic legend in an occupational sub-culture. In: Dingwall R, McIntosh J 1978 Readings in the sociology of nursing. Churchill Livingstone, Edinburgh

Wilding P 1982 Professional Power and social welfare. Routledge & Kegan Paul, London

FURTHER READING

Curtin L, Flaherty M J 1982 Nursing ethics, theories and pragmatics, Robert J Brady Maryland

Davis A J Aroskar M A 1978 Ethical dilemmas and nursing practice. Appleton Century Crofts, New York

Faulder C 1985 Whose body is it? The troubled issue of informed consent, Virago, London

Kohnke M F 1982 Advocacy: Risk and reality, C V Mosby St Louis, Miss.

4

Power-sharing and personal values in nursing ethics

4.1 Models of power relationships and the origins of ethics

In a fundamental sense ethics is concerned with power and power relationships. It is concerned both with how we exercise power and authority over other people, and how we exercise responsibility and care for other people. However, it is also concerned with our personal striving to fulfil our potential as human beings. Ethics is not simply other-related, but also about our own personal fulfilment. If ethics is about how we share power in human communities, then it is also about how we protect one another's rights and promote one another's well-being. An egocentric ethics will place the emphasis on my right to fulfil my potential, my powers of being as a person. An altruistic ethics will tend to sacrifice self-interest in the service of others. (Tillich 1954, Campbell 1984.)

In practice, nursing ethics needs to maintain a balance between the two. Job satisfaction and personal fulfilment in a nursing career are important ethically, for without adequate emphasis on the needs of the nurse the quality of patient care will suffer, and frustration and poor staff morale will undermine competence and efficiency in the service. On the other hand, selfless service in the care and treatment of others, respecting their dignity and value as human beings, gives satisfaction to work, however menial. Mere careerism, or the attitude of 'it's just another job', deprives nursing of professional dignity if other-regarding values of care are neglected. However, some forms of care can be dependency-creating, turning people into perennial 'patients', if nursing care is not directed to empower patients to 'stand on their own feet again', and to restore autonomy, where possible, to people who have lost it as a consequence of illness, injury or mental disorder. Thus the ethics of nursing, like that of other 'caring professions', is fundamentally about power relationships and power sharing (Campbell 1985).

There are various ways we can analyse the forms in which power and responsibility exercised in health care have a bearing on our understanding of nursing ethics. A *sociological analysis* will focus attention on the structure of power relationships in different social settings — e.g. in consulting relationships, in the home, in institutional settings, in more public and political contexts — and will analyse the different ways moral values and personal or professional responsibility are interpreted in each situation. Each social setting will be governed by its own set of formal and informal rules. A *philosophical analysis* will focus more on the logical relationships between the fundamental principles which embody our basic moral values, and the practical criteria we use in making moral judgements and applying our principles to concrete situations which demand decisions from us. From a philosophical point of view we appeal to fundamental moral principles to legitimate our exercise of power, and to define its responsible use. An *historical analysis* will look at the evolution of a given society (or societies) and will seek to describe the way values have developed in the creation of its institutions and specialised roles in the division of labour. Thus, in relation to health care it will examine the development of medical science and traditions of medical practice; related developments of nursing functions in lay, religious, military, hospital and community settings; and the ethical codes evolved in each profession. As the emergence of different professions has been marked by the formal differentiation of roles and demarcation of different areas of responsibility or functions within health care, so each has developed its own peculiar set of values.

While we recognise that a great deal could be written, and has been written, about the history of health care and the nursing profession (Abel-Smith 1960, Freidson 1970, White 1970, Ehrenreich & English 1973, Davies 1979), in this chapter we will discuss mainly sociological and philosophical models for interpreting moral issues in health care, and in nursing ethics in particular. As the sociological and philosophical analyses draw much of their material from the history of ideas and the general history of culture, the historical dimensions of the subject are not being ignored and are implicit in much of what follows. Thus the historical development in Western society of particular institutions and models of practice in health care is relevant to a proper understanding of how we perceive professional–client relationships today. It is also directly relevant to understanding the respective rights and duties of professionals and their clients and the values which govern their relationships with one another.

4.2 Models for the ethics of carer–client relationships

In his now famous book Illich (1977) put forward a wealth of historical evidence to demonstrate that over the past 150 years the medical profession has come to exercise increasing control over our lives, from birth to death. This process of the so-called 'medicalisation of life' is reflected in several developments related to 'medical imperialism': increasing professionalisation of health care; expansion of medical services into new territories, traditionally the domain of lay care (e.g. bereavement counselling, sex therapy); growing dependence of lay people on medical 'experts' for help, with corresponding loss of skills and confidence among lay people; increasing institutionalisation of health care.

This process, which has been confirmed in research by other historians and social scientists, has profound implications for the way we understand the ethics of health care. It has already led in the last decade to major new initiatives in health education and public health promotion, not least by the World Health Organisation (WHO 1978, 1979, 1981), to attempt to reverse this process, and to encourage the confidence and competence of lay people to take responsibility for their own health. However, it is still the dominant reality in most countries. The fact is that the vast majority of mothers in Europe have their babies delivered in hospital rather than at home; that mentally handicapped people and those who are mentally ill tend to be kept in special mental hospitals; that people attend special clinics for problems connected with drug and alcohol abuse, obesity, family planning, sexual problems and stress; and the overwhelming majority of people now die in hospital or in special terminal care units, whereas a century ago these problems would have been dealt with at home or in the community. This process, and in particular the institutionalisation of health care, brings its own special complications to the discussion of ethical issues in nursing or health care generally.

There are subtle and important differences between the ethics of different situations and settings in health care. Professional ethics in primary care or community settings differs in important respects from that which governs relationships in hospitals or other institutions (Freidson 1970, Thompson 1979). Different rules and constraints operate in each case. Yet other rules govern managerial, policy-making and political roles in the health professions, making the ethics of these domains different again. This is not to say that the fundamental principles and values are not the same, but the problems and constraints, rules and forms of accountability, do vary considerably with the exercise of power and responsibility in each of these different kinds of situations.

In this and the preceding discussion we have made use of four key concepts which are derived from sociological analysis of caring relationships, but which are very important and useful in philosophical analysis of ethics too. These concepts are: Situations, Roles, Rules and Arbiters. (Emmet 1966, Thompson 1979).

It may seem obvious that the nurse meets patients or clients in a variety of different kinds of situations. However, it is not always so obvious that the nurse's role in each of these situations may be different, that the rules of practice defining duties and responsibilities in each situation may be different, and that the nurse will be accountable to different people who act as arbiters of the nurse's performance in each different context. It is the aim of the next two sections to explore a number of different models for caring and management relationships, to demonstrate how roles, rules and arbiters change in different professional settings or situations.

Code, contract and covenant

Consider for example the nurse as a member of a *crisis intervention* team (in accident and emergency, intensive care, in emergency obstetrics, or acute medical, surgical or psychiatric units). This situation differs in important respects from situations where the nurse is involved in a *consulting role* (giving advice on family planning, antenatal or post-natal care, interviewing or assessing competent adult patients, or in making domiciliary visits in a monitoring, advisory, supportive or clinical capacity). A third type of situation, which differs in significant respects from the other two, is where the nurse is responsible for *continuity-of-care* in a long-term or chronic situation (in care of severely mentally handicapped persons, patients with chronic mental or physical illness, in geriatric nursing, terminal care and support of the bereaved).

In these three different situations of crisis intervention, consultation and continuity of care in chronic illness, professional ethics tends to be governed by three different kinds of models, namely: code-based, contractual, and covenantal ethics respectively. Let us examine each of these models in turn, considering what special values or ethical principles underlie them.

Historically, each of the caring professions in formulating its professional ethics has tended to do so first in terms of a *code of practice*. These in turn tend to be preoccupied with consideration of what the duties of professionals are when they are required to intervene in a crisis, particularly where the client or patient (sufferer) is unconscious or unconsultable, or incompetent because of youth, senility or mental disorder. On the one hand codes tend to justify crisis interventions by carers in terms of their duty to care for the vulnerable and incompetent and to protect them from harm (the principle of beneficence or non-maleficence). On the other hand, because the carer is in charge and has responsibility for the well-being of the person committed to their care, codes also seek to prevent malpractice and to protect carers from unfair claims or demands being made on them by those for whom they have provided care (or their representatives). The law and ethics may often speak of the carer as acting in such situations '*in loco parentis*' (in place of the parent) or '*parens patriae*' (as a parent on behalf of the state). This quasiparental protective beneficence, or duty-to-care, carries with it the risk of becoming patronising and of creating and perpetuating dependency in the patient or client, exemplified by the phrase 'doctor/nurse knows best'. It has become fashionable to criticise patronising professional attitudes and practices which tend to 'infantilise' people, compromise their dignity and disregard their rights. However, we cannot completely dispense with protective beneficence as a professional value or personal virtue, as we are all extremely vulnerable at certain times in our lives. We will always need others to help and protect us when we are weak and vulnerable, and to defend our rights when we are unable to do so ourselves.

In the client-initiated consultation, the client voluntarily approaches the carer with some problem, seeking help. The carer is assumed to have the knowledge, skills or access to resources to give the necessary help. The carer, in offering a service, is involved in direct negotiation with the client about the nature and scope of the help required and, in the process, establishes either a formal or informal *contract-to-care*. The client, in voluntarily entrusting himself into the care of the carer, accepts the responsibility to co-operate with the carer in the help given, e.g. by giving relevant personal details, allowing physical examination or other kinds of tests and assessments to be made. The carer accepts the duty to respect the trust shown by the client by providing a competent service, protecting the patient's dignity and observing the requirements of confidentiality. This contractual relationship, like other commercial and legal contracts, is governed by the demands of natural justice and recognition of mutual rights and duties. Although the relationship between the person-with-the-problem and the person-with-the-power-to-help is an inherently unequal one, the same is likely to be true of any relationship with a plumber or motor-mechanic from whom you seek help. However, these situations are different from those where one is completely helpless and/or given help without being consulted. The fiduciary responsibility (from Latin *fiducia*, trust) of the carer is based on the fact that the client entrusts themselves into the hands of the carer and agrees to bear the cost of that commitment (and does not default on payment — where this is appropriate). The carers' responsibility to perform their service to the best of their ability, with knowledge, skill and consideration of the clients' rights and interests, and not to abuse or exploit them, is obviously a requirement of justice.

In order to clarify what we mean by personal rights (particularly the rights of patients or clients) it is instructive to consider the third type of situation, because in situations of chronic or terminal illness these appear in their most poignant form. In providing continuity-of-care in situations of long-term or chronic illness, particularly where there is no hope of cure but only amelioration of symptoms, a different kind of commitment on both sides is required. Where the patient is competent and consultable, there may be a need to renegotiate the contract-to-care. Where the presuppositions of the original contract-to-care are based on therapeutic optimism, the expectation is that the carer has the necessary knowledge, skills and therapeutic resources to help. If this situation changes so that the client's condition is chronic or deteriorating, and the carer can offer only palliative care or personal support, then the nature of the new situation ought to be acknowledged. The client has a particular right to know, to accept or refuse the new regimen of palliative care, and the right to appropriate privacy in negotiations about these matters. The carer, on the other hand, has a duty to make clear what is being offered. If this is emotional and spiritual support, counselling or just a commitment to 'care to the end', this should be understood on both sides.

Such a new kind of caring relationship, based on a commitment of mutual fidelity, requires a different name. May (1975) suggested *covenant*, following the Biblical meaning. If 'care' is not to be officiously given, or continued without due regard for the patient's views or personal rights; and if the patient is to be prevented from becoming more dependent and either parasitic upon or exploitative of the care given, then despite the vulnerability of the patient, the scope and nature of the continuing caring relationship needs to be reviewed and renegotiated. The principle of respect for persons, which underlies this concept of covenantal ethics is not only concerned with protecting the rights and dignity of the patient or client, but ultimately those of the carer as well. If the supererogatory duties are not to become a burden or a means of exploitation, then they have to be accepted freely by the carer in gratitude for the trust and affection shown by the patient.

The principles of beneficence, justice, and respect for persons, which underlie these three models, are not mutually exclusive but complementary, though there may be tensions between them at different times. Just as there are areas of overlap between the three different kinds of situations, so there are interconnections between beneficence, justice and respect for persons. In crisis intervention, beneficence has to be complemented by considerations of justice and respect for persons, if its exercise is not to lead to patronising attitudes to 'patients', and practices which create chronic dependency in them. In the voluntarily negotiated contract-to-care the client may still need to be protected, as, for example, beneficence demands that the professional respects the patient's right to properly informed consent, and strict justice may have to be compromised as attention to the special needs of people with acute conditions may result in less attention being given to other people's needs. Conversely, special regard for the needs and rights of individuals has to be balanced by consideration of the common good, as in the case where patients may have to be quarantined to protect others in an epidemic. Here justice and respect for the rights of individuals may appear to be in conflict in the exercise of the general duty to care.

Command, critical enquiry and community responsibility

There is another group of situations in which nurses or other health professionals are involved when they move out of direct patient-care into management, teaching and research, and the exercise of community responsibility in more public and 'political' roles. Here the models which are applicable become more complex and various, but we may possibly discuss them under three different headings: Command, Critical enquiry, and Community responsibility.

Command. The exercise of power and responsibility in management roles is tied up with the concept of authority (from Latin *augere*, to implement or augment). To exercise authority you must be authorised by some person or body of persons to hold some official post to carry out some official function. Authority in this sense means legitimate power — power legitimated by election, official selection or promotion, or direct appointment by higher authority. To exercise authority also means to exercise power in such a way that you work to promote the well-being of those over whom you have 'authority', not just to promote your own interest or those of the institution. Thus the naked or dictatorial exercise of power offends against the duty to care, the requirements of natural justice and respect for persons under your authority.

Management styles can vary and so can models of management. Line-management, or a straight chain of command, is the official structure within the nursing hierarchy. This corresponds to the pattern of management in large institutions, or to the requirements of management in situations of crisis such as war or medical, surgical and psychiatric emergencies. However, team management, with shared authority and responsibility, may be more appropriate in other areas, as is becoming evident in primary care, rehabilitation, and long-term care of medical and psychiatric patients. Personal management styles may vary from a controlling style to permissive, directive to democratic, authoritarian to consensus-based.

It is not our purpose to discuss the advantages or disadvantages of the different models or styles of management, but rather to stress that each embodies certain values and is based on different formal and informal rules. Roles will be different within each system, as well as the formal and informal rules which obtain, and expectations about who is responsible ('carries the can') and to whom officers are accountable ('who will blame me if things go wrong').

Traditional line-management invests considerable power in those at the top, who, it is assumed, will exercise power responsibly in a just and beneficent way, even though they may be employed with a specific mandate to improve efficiency and to make savings. Thus, for example, if there have to be staff cuts, it is assumed that these will not be made capriciously but in a way that is fair, protects the wider interests of the service, does not discriminate against particular groups, and has due regard to the statutory rights of employees. Alternatively, in a more democratic style of team management on the ward or in the community, the values of respect for persons have high priority. This should apply to the respect between people of different professional background in regard for one another's expertise, sharing of work and responsibility, and of information about patients or clients. It should also be reflected in the style of interaction with patients or clients and in respect for their rights.

Critical enquiry. All professions base their claim to special status and regard in the eyes of other professions and the public on their mastery of certain knowledge and skills, and responsibility for the disposal and administration of certain public resources (Freidson 1970). Therefore, education and training play an important part in the preparation of professionals for their work, serving both as a basis for their power and as a means to legitimate their claims to expertise, whether in helping others or in performing some function. The responsibility of a profession to maintain the highest possible standards in education and training is not just about maintaining status and power, but perhaps more fundamentally it is a requirement of justice to provide a competent and efficient service for the benefit of their clients and society as a whole.

However, education and training are not of much value if they perpetuate bad practice, if they are never properly evaluated. Thus teaching and research are integrally related, in the interests of ensuring the competence and efficiency of staff and the service as a whole, and the most effective and cost-efficient care for clients and patients. Not only the financial cost but the human cost should be considered, thus raising questions of respect for persons and their rights. In comparative evaluation of the cost efficiency of different procedures or management practices, again not only are considerations of an economic nature relevant but also the common good of patients.

Specific ethical issues in teaching and research are discussed in Chapter 8, but the point of raising them here is that critical enquiry is a necessary part of the function of any profession. Competent and efficient care is a requirement of beneficence, in the protection of clients from malpractice, and it is not possible without sound education and training, and scientific research on and validation of professional practice. Truthfulness is not only about honesty and sharing information with clients, it is also about scientific integrity, rigour in enquiry, and honesty in the publication of results for the benefit of all — a requirement of justice. Knowledge and skills acquired in training are meant to be shared with clients and used to assist them back to health and greater independence. The use of training in responsible care and rehabilitation of those who seek help is both a requirement of beneficence and respect for their right to autonomy as persons.

Community responsibility. To be a professional means that, by definition, one exercises a public role, a public office. It is therefore impossible for professionals to ignore their duty of accountability to the wider community, without ceasing to be responsible professionals. In this sense all professionals have a political role in addition to the particular function which they perform in the division of labour. Nurses, especially those in senior positions, take on public and 'political' roles in many situations. They may be involved in committees for a variety of purposes: administrative, planning, research anad training. They may be involved in professional associations, trade unions, government advisory and policy-making bodies, or interprofessional, interagency, or international committees. They may be involved in community nursing and community health in promoting self-help groups, community development projects and community action, or even in direct political action at local, regional or national level.

The skilful, effective and morally sound exercise of community responsibility has to be learned, like anything else. While people are given management training and taught to teach and do research, most skills associated with the exercise of power in these more public and political roles for nurses, have to be learned by experience. Working on committees may be less glamorous than nursing patients;

campaigning for higher professional standards or better patient care, through professional bodies, unions or pressure groups, may seem remote from direct patient care; community development and community action may seem to mix nursing and politics, but all these activities are relevant to nursing ethics. Ethics and politics are never totally separate or separable, but continuous with one another, as Aristotle recognised 2000 years ago (Thomson 1953). Personal responsibility and professional responsibility mix ethics and politics, for all professionals should be publicly accountable. Health care cannot be simply about the alleviation of individual distress but the common weal — as it is about the rights and dignity of individuals and the common good, about individual health promotion and Health For All By the Year 2000.

4.3 Historical and cultural diversity and common ethical principles

In the general study of ethics we set out to study the underlying principles common to all types of personal and social morality. But are we justified in assuming that there are common underlying principles?

We often hear it said, 'When it comes to morality everyone seems to have different views of what is right and wrong'. And 'Who are we to say that one person is right and another wrong?' We also are becoming aware that we live in a world where the great religions of Islam, Hinduism, Buddhism, Judaism and Christianity, as well as secular ideologies such as Marxism and Humanism, seem to be competing for the allegiance of men and women — offering them different systems of values and different means of salvation. In Britain and in other European countries with a colonial past, colonial expansion brought contact and sometimes conflict with other cultural and religious traditions. In this century, global wars and revolutions have created huge refugee populations, social upheaval and dislocation, affecting millions of people. This change, coupled with global trade, travel, emigration and immigration, has left few cultures unchallenged by interaction with others. The reality is that few of us live any longer in isolated or culturally homogenous societies. Britain itself is a multicultural society (and perhaps always has been), and is increasingly a multi-ethnic society too. The National Health Service not only has to deal with clients from an incredible variety of religious, political and cultural backgrounds, but its staff represents the same variety and diversity too. On the one hand, this diversity and confusing variety of traditions of religious and social morality seems to make the talk of common principles seem naive and moral consensus an unrealistic dream. On the other hand, if we are not over-whelmed by the relativities and driven to moral scepticism, we can only wonder at the richness and variety of forms in which human beings have sought to express what they believe it means to be human and what values they see to be necessary to make possible a full life (Veatch 1981).

Moral relativism and scepticism are useful challenges to thinking about ethics. As the German philosopher Kant pointed out in the eighteenth century, when we say that something is right or wrong we are making an implicit or explicit claim that this is, or should be, true for everybody (Paton 1969). This claim to universal validity implicit in ordinary moral judgements is challenged by the evidence of moral disagreements between individuals and the diversity of moral rules in different systems of social morality. In the face of scepticism based on moral relativism, namely that all moral beliefs are relative, relative either to the individual or his culture, we are driven to find more fundamental principles which underlie these apparent individual and cultural differences.

The challenge represented by moral scepticism is to provide some kind of rational justification for these fundamental principles, once we have found them. The rational debate about the foundations of ethics as such takes us into the sphere of moral theory — a subject we will return to in the final chapter. We can pursue the demand for rational justification for moral principles only so far as is reasonable. If nothing will satisfy us but absolute certainty, then perhaps nothing will satisfy us, and we are left with paralysing scepticism. In practice, we do manage to get along more or less well with people of other religious and cultural traditions and we share enough common ground to do business with one another, intermarry, and even vote for the same political parties. Moral scepticism has to make sense of this creative interaction between widely different human cultures, or it simply leads to a kind of cul-de-sac of thought and action.

For some people, the quest for the foundations of morality leads back to metaphysical beliefs about the nature of ultimate reality, or to religion and beliefs about God and immortality. Historically, most systems of social morality have evolved from metaphysical and religious beliefs, and it is always interesting, and often instructive, to trace their pedigree. However, it can be argued that ethics can, or should be, able to stand without the supports of religion and metaphysics, that it should be able to stand on the basis of rational criteria like comprehensiveness, coherence and consistency, and congruence with our experience of what it means to be human. For many people on the other hand, those who are less bothered by sceptical doubts, the matter is more pragmatic — how to reconcile their moral beliefs with those of others in such a way that conflict can be avoided or reduced and co-operation made possible (Maritain 1964).

If we are to avoid giving unnecessary offence or injuring other people's moral sensibilities, we need to develop tolerance and an understanding, even respect, for moral standpoints which differ from our own. This is not easy. We are born into particular families and societies, with their own unique traditions and values. Commitment to these values and willingness to live by them, fight for them, and in some cases to die for them, is a vital source of cohesion and solidarity in families and communities. Also, such values serve to define our identity as members of such social groups. For children born of parents of widely different cultural and religious views or ethnic origin, the conflict of values can be both painful and a source of enrichment. For people working in the caring professions, awareness of cultural and religious differences is not only important for dealing with confusion or disagreements of a moral nature, but may be vital in understanding what factors (dress, diet, genetic differences, customs relating to birth, reproduction and death) are directly relevant to their physical and mental health.

At a broader level, Christianity, Marxism, and Islam, as three great 'religions', have sent out missionaries to spread these respective 'gospels' and to make converts. In the course of their endeavours they have often treated with contempt

the traditional religion and customs of the societies they have penetrated. At best, they have been guilty of a kind of cultural imperialism — the arrogant and often self-righteous claim to proprietorship of the truth or of privileged access to moral wisdom. At worst, they have been guilty of forced conversions, witchhunts, persecution and suppression of religious practices other than their own. Against this, the painstaking studies of anthopologists and sociologists and the cross-cultural comparisons made on the basis of more objective and scientific analyses have not only brought to light the diversity and relativity of social customs and mores, but have also helped us to gain insight into the rich wisdom and dignity of many cultures we might be tempted to call primitive.

Moral relativism has therefore helped to challenge cultural imperialism, religious and moral dogmatism, intolerance and arrogance. However, it must also be pointed out that there have been thinkers and leaders among Christians, Marxists and Muslims, who have also criticised these tendencies among their co-religionists or party supporters. For Christians it has been in the name of a god who transcends and judges all human institutions. For some Marxists it has been in the name of a science which is experimental and tentative, not dogmatic, and recognition of the need for ongoing reform even after the Russian Revolution. For the great philosophers of Islam, it has been in the name of an uncompromising ethical monotheism, and a belief in universal human values. The recognition of some kind of transcendent ideal itself may be grounds for a kind of moral relativism — the humility to recognise the limited and fallible nature of our own moral systems or personal insights.

The argument based on moral relativism can, however, be so exaggerated as to make nonsense of moral argument and the reality of human intercultural co-operation. If there were no common ground between the moral beliefs of different individuals or different peoples, then rational debate and intelligent disagreement about ethical and political concerns would not be possible. The reality is that even people with the most widely divergent views continue to debate moral principles and values in a way that they do not do about mere matters of taste (*de gustibus non est disputandum*). This suggests that there is sufficient common ground for each disputant to at least understand (or partially understand) what the other is saying, and thus attempt to marshal arguments, feelings, and evidence in the effort to persuade the other. The reality is that throughout history diverse nations and cultures have been able to form pacts and alliances, co-operate in peace and war, and even develop the basis of public and international law. The United Nations Declaration of Human Rights (UNO 1948), although not signed by the USSR and South Africa in 1947, was nevertheless signed by the official representatives of all other member states. The further elaboration of this Bill of Rights and the growing body of international law, and the enhanced authority of the International Court of Human Rights, suggest that there is in fact more agreement about fundamental principles and human rights than might at first sight be apparent from the seemingly interminable wrangles in public debate and in forums such as the European Parliament or the United Nations General Assembly (Cowen 1961).

This should not altogether surprise us, for, despite the seemingly infinite variety of human beings and forms of social and political organisation, some things are universally common to all members of our species. For example, in all human societies children are born through the fertilisation of sperm and ovum from parents of different sex; children are born very small and vulnerable — needing to be fed, nurtured and protected. With luck, good management and effective health care they may survive the infections and traumas of childhood; may reach maturity, reproduce themselves, decline into old age and sooner or later all will die. These universal features of human life suggest that there are bound to be features of all systems of social morality which are similar. If certain general conditions must be satisfied before human life can develop and flourish, then there will have to be general principles of morality which seek to protect vulnerable human life and promote these conditions for human flourishing (d'Entreves 1964).

This question can be approached in two different ways: either by attempting to define the essential conditions which must be satisfied if human life is to be human, which leads to the formulation of *fundamental human rights*; or by attempting to clarify the fundamental values by which we seek to direct human action and social organisation to protect human beings and to promote human flourishing, which leads to the formulation of *fundamental principles*.

4.4 Fundamental human rights and common principles of ethics

Attempts to formulate universal human rights go back to antiquity. The Stoics believed that the natural world is a rationally ordered cosmos, not a meaningless chaos. This rational order which they observed (in the movements of the sun, moon and stars, in the cycle of the seasons, the phenomena of growth and decay, the processes of change in inorganic matter, and the ordered character of human society) had to have its origin, they argued, in a macrocosmic order of divine origin. The microcosmic order of the human mind was in these terms just a scaled down and imperfect version of this divine rational order. The Stoics sought to ground the rationality and universality of human laws in the 'natural laws' of the cosmos, and to ground universal human rights in the essential nature of man as a rational being.

This faith in man as a rational animal, part of a rational universe, inspired the pragmatic 'natural law' principles which the Roman and medieval jurists applied (in theory at least) to people of all kinds and different cultures without discrimination. Although the Romans distinguished between the special laws applicable to Roman citizens and the *'jus gentium'*, or law applied to all others, both were supposed to be grounded in certain principles of natural justice, the *'jus naturale'*. Ordinary citizens could appeal to the principles of natural justice against unjust laws or in seeking to defend their rights. The great Dutch legal theorists of the seventeenth century (such as Grotius) who adapted the principles of natural law to modern use are the fathers of the kinds of bills of rights adopted by the leaders of the French and American revolutions, which find their developed expression in modern public and international law and the United Nations Universal Declaration of Human Rights. The difference between the classical and modern theories of natural law, as the basis of individual human rights, consists mainly in the fact that the former believed natural law to be inherent in the nature of the cosmos itself, the latter that it is derived more from the demands of social organisation, social contracts and conventions. (Scots Law to this day retains important elements of this Roman/Dutch legal tradition.) (Cowen 1961, d'Entreves 1964.)

Bills of rights tend to be constructed on arguments of the following kind:

if we can say that being human means having the following essential attributes or capacities—rational intelligence (Greek and Roman), capacity to love (Judeo-Christian), or capacity for creative work (Marxism);

then it follows that individual human beings must have certain rights — freedom of expression, freedom of association, freedom of movement — to ensure that they are able to develop and express their human attributes and natural capacities.

Thus the right to freedom of speech, freedom of association, freedom of political or religious affiliation and perhaps freedom of movement too could be said to be necessary conditions for human beings to develop their potentialities as rational beings. While the emphasis on rational intelligence as the primary defining characteristic of human beings has been the dominant tradition in Western culture, it is not the only tradition: the Judeo–Christian and Marxist traditions emphasise other human attributes and correspondingly different human rights. A consequence of our cultural bias towards the definition of essential humanity in terms of rational intelligence is that we place a high premium on IQ and educational achievement as well as scientific knowledge, but it also means that we devalue those people with low intelligence and, characteristically, the mentally handicapped and mentally ill tend to be relegated to the margins of society and to suffer neglect. These areas of health care have especially low status.

Emphasis on the capacity to love and on social interaction and co-operation leads on to other rights of a more social and political nature — for instance, rights to privacy, domicile, and nationality, to participation in government in addition to freedom of speech, movement and association. While the Judeo-Christian emphasis on love and social interaction is an important corrective to the emphasis on intelligence alone, it can also lead to lack of sympathy for those who are lacking in social skills or who are emotionally deprived and perhaps pathologically incapable of love or personal warmth.

The stress in Marxism on the capacity for creative work, the capacity to apply one's brain and one's hands to transform the material and social environment, highlights the importance of work to individuals as a means for developing their physical and mental capacities as well as building social links through co-operation. Marxism has stressed the right to work, the right to just rewards for one's labour, freedom from exploitation or enslavement, together with other political rights such as freedom of immigration/emigration to seek employment (Veatch 1981).

It is perhaps too easy to suggest that each of these traditions emphasises complementary aspects of what it means to be human, for over the centuries much blood has been shed in the defence of rights which have been given priority within one social system or another. The Universal Declaration of Human Rights adopted and proclaimed by the General Assembly of the United Nations Organisation on 10 December 1948, inevitably combined features from these and other traditions and a compromise between them. It did not attempt to define which rights are primary and fundamental and which are derivative, but to suggest that the rights to personal freedom and equality (especially equality before the law and equality of opportunity) are fundamental, or perhaps summed up in Article 3: 'Everyone has the right to life, liberty and security of person.' (The American Constitution has it as 'the right to life, liberty and the pursuit of happiness'). Of course, many other rights flow from these, and the UN Declaration includes the right to freedom from discrimination on grounds of race, religion, sex, etc. (Article 2, 3) and the rights to education and adequate health care (Articles 25 and 26) (UNO 1948).

However, the more these rights are elaborated the more we become aware of other principles which have a constitutive and regulative function in relation to the organisation of social life. If it is true that in all societies people are born, grow to maturity, may reproduce, grow old and die, then it is also inevitable that the *constitutive and regulative principles* of life within a moral community will bear some resemblance to one another from one society to the next. These commonalities of human life are sufficient to explain how all societies and human families, however structured, recognise the quasi-parental *duty-to-care* — for children, the weak, the sick and the vulnerable. As individuals grow to maturity and seek to negotiate on their own behalf and to participate in society, so the demands for liberty, equality, fraternity — the demands of public justice — begin to emerge, often challenging patronising beneficence. As individuals emerge in the family or society with greater power and ability to exercise independent moral responsibility, particularly as the roles are reversed with the assumption of authority by the new generation, respect for the autonomy and dignity of persons as persons becomes a more central issue.

Simple clan or tribal society, monarchies and hierarchical societies (including religious orders and the traditional professions of law and medicine) have organised around the exacting of a duty of obedience from members or clients in return for the assurance of some kind of protective *beneficence*. The more rational organisation required by urban civilisation has led, as in Greek and Roman culture, to a greater emphasis on public *justice* and the rights and duties which go with membership of the civic order, particularly for free men. The emphasis in Judeo-Christian religion on the unique dignity of each individual 'in the sight of God' has highlighted *respect for persons* as the primary demand of an ethic of love. Elements of these three principles — beneficence, justice and respect for persons — can be found in the ethical traditions of all human societies, even though particular historical communities may tend to emphasise the primacy of one rather than the other.

Socialist societies may tend, for example, to stress the primacy of social justice and the protective duty-to-care of the state, with less emphasis on or actual compromise of individual rights. Self-styled liberal democracies give primacy to individual liberty and personal rights, but these cannot be guaranteed or protected without complementary emphasis on social justice and the duty to care for the vulnerable. The principle of protective beneficence, or the duty to care, is paramount in all social structures where powerful individuals rule over weaker people, in family and tribal life and in more traditional systems of monarchic government. For the same reason, the health and caring professions have tended to emphasise the duty to care as the primary organising principle of their service to clients and patients. Considerations of justice tend to come in later in public health, prevention of disease, planning, research and management — where concern with groups rather than individuals becomes more important. Concern with individual rights tends to evolve at a later stage, often in response to criticism by clients or patients of the patronising 'doctor/nurse knows best' maxim. The importance of the principles of respect of persons, justice and beneficence as fundamental ethical principles can be demonstrated in another way too, which derives from philosophical reflection on the nature of ethical systems and what principles are logically necessary for their construction (Beauchamp & Childress 1979).

4.5 Constitutive and regulative principles of ethics

In his *Groundwork to the methaphysic of morals* (1785) the German philosopher Immanuel Kant argued that the concept of Person or Personhood, is fundamental to ethics (Paton 1969). Without the concept of a person — an individual who is a bearer of rights and responsibilities — ethics cannot get started. Such individuals must always be treated as ends in themselves and never simply as instrumental means to an end. Thus the concept of a person is one of the constitutive principles of ethics, and serves to define the membership and scope of the moral community. In excluding the exploitation or abuse of persons, the *principle of respect for persons* also serves as a practical and regulative principle of social conduct.

However, the concept of a person, or even a derived list of personal rights, would not alone be sufficient to establish a coherent system of ethics. Personal rights alone would not provide an adequate basis for a system of social ethics unless these rights could be justified, promoted and protected as rights for all. This requires a principle of universalisability, as Kant called it, to ensure that individuals act consistently and that the rights claimed for individuals are applied to all without discrimination. This demand for equity or universal fairness, is really a demand of the *principle of justice*.

Justice and respect for persons together would make for a

reasonably satisfactory combination of pillars for any system of ethics but for the fact of given inequalities — the fact that there are wide discrepancies of size and age, wealth and power, intelligence and skill, health and strength among human beings. To ensure a workable system of ethics we require another principle, which we might call the principle of reciprocity ('Do unto others as you would have them do unto you'). This principle is necessary because at certain times in our lives we are extremely vulnerable, when we are infants, sick, injured, mentally disordered, senile or dying. Unless we build in a principle of reciprocity — the recognition of a reciprocal duty to care for one another — we cannot ground the social obligation to care for or protect the interests of the weak. The *principle of beneficence* (the duty to care, or to do good) and the principle of non-maleficence (the duty to do no harm to those in your care) thus complement respect for personal rights and justice, and complete the minimum requirements for a coherent system of ethics.

In the context of health care, respect for persons basically means treating patients as persons with rights. It means further respecting the autonomy of individuals and protecting those who suffer loss of autonomy through illness, injury or mental disorder, and working to restore autonomy to those who have lost it. It means recognising that patients have such basic human rights as the right to know, the right to privacy and the right to receive care and treatment. Clearly, there may be a tension between the patient's rights and the helper's duty to care, just as there may be practical difficulties in determining adequately informed and voluntary consent to treatment; or in setting sensible limits to confidentiality, or physical privacy, in institutions where care may be shared by a team of nurses, paramedics, social workers and doctors; and distinguishing between care and treatment or the choice of therapies. For the carers, respect for persons in their care means working to maintain the optimum degree of independence for the patient, and sharing knowledge, care and skills in such a way as to avoid creating and perpetuating dependency (Henderson 1964, Ramsey 1970, RCN 1979).

Justice, or the demand for universal fairness, stands in a relationship of tension with respect for persons. The exercise of individual rights (such as freedom of movement or association) may have to be limited in the interests of the common good, as in cases where public health measures have to be introduced to contain epidemics. In this context we are not really concerned with retributive but with distributive justice, but the restriction of individual liberties may appear punitive to infected individuals — for example, the way AIDS sufferers have been treated in some societies is reminiscent of past treatment of lepers or the mentally ill. When we consider the social controls imposed on the mentally disordered and the loss of rights of people in institutional care generally, or the policing role which nurses and other health care workers may have to perform, the analogy with retributive justice seems close (as the sociological analysis of sickness behaviour as a kind of deviance illustrates) (Freidson 1970). However justified public health measures may be, we must not lose sight of the rights of individuals. Justice to individuals also means non-discrimination on the basis of sex, race, religion, etc. (or because of youth, old age, having a contagious disease, mental handicap or mental illness). It means equal opportunity to benefit from, or have access to, preventive medicine and treatment health services and to the benefits of research. Justice also means equality of outcomes for groups, and relates to the broader 'political' responsibilities of health professionals in controlling and allocating resources, in planning, research and development. The evidence in the Black Report (Townsend & Davidson 1982) and in the Health Education Council's report (Whitehead 1987) demonstrates that to ensure justice in health care political action may be required to shift greater resources to deprived areas at the expense of more privileged sectors. Campaigning for resources to improve services or to defend standards of care are both requirements laid on health professionals by the demands of the principles of justice.

Beneficence has had a bad press recently. Attacks on medical paternalism and resentment of the medicalisation of life, the emphasis on patients' rights by militant pressure groups, action by politicians concerned with social justice and the political economy of health care have resulted in health professionals becoming defensive about beneficence. Certainly, beneficence, the duty to care, may be exercised in a way that 'infantilises' people and creates dependence, but it need not do so. In fact, it has been argued that patient advocacy, defending the rights of the vulnerable patient, is a requirement of beneficence. Beneficence is indispensable wherever there are dependent or helpless people in need of support or urgent care and attention. The reciprocity in our duty to care for one another should make us realise that we all need others to speak for us, to do things for us, when we are too weak to do so for ourselves. But if knowledge is power, the power of the true carer is aimed at sharing knowledge and skills with the vulnerable individual so as to empower that person to reassert control over their own life, if this is humanly possible. (May 1983, Campbell 1984, 1985.)

REFERENCES

Abel-Smith B 1960 A history of the nursing profession, Heinemann, London
Beauchamp T, Childress J 1979 Principles of bio-medical ethics. Oxford University Press
Campbell A V 1984 Moderated love. SPCK, London, Ch 2, 3
Campbell A V 1985 Paid to care. SPCK, London
Cowen D 1961 The foundations of freedom. Oxford University Press
Davies C 1979 Rewriting nursing history. Croom Helm, Beckenham
d'Entreves A 1964 Natural Law. Hutchinson, London
Ehrenreich B, English D 1973 Witches, midwives and nurses: A history of women healers. Readers and Writers Cooperative, London
Emmet D 1966 Rules, roles and relations. Macmillan, London
Freidson E 1970 Profession of medicine. Dodd Mead, New York
Henderson V 1964 The nature of nursing. American Journal of Nursing 64, 63
Illich I 1977 The limits of medicine. Medical nemesis: The expropriation of health. Penguin Books, Harmondsworth
Maritain J 1964 Moral philosophy. Bles, London, Ch 1–3, 5
May W 1975 Code, Covenant, Contract or Philanthropy. Hastings Center Report No 5
May W 1983 The Physician's Covenant. Westminster, Philadelphia
Paton H J (trans.) 1969 The Moral Law: Kant's groundwork of the metaphysics of morals. Bles, London
Ramsey P 1970 The patient as person. Yale University Press, New Haven, Conn.
Royal College of Nursing 1979 Code of Professional Conduct: Discussion document. RCN, London
Thompson I 1979 Dilemmas of dying — A study in the ethics of terminal care, Edinburgh University Press, Edinburgh
Thompson I E 1987 Fundamental ethical principles in health care. British Medical Journal, 295 5 December 1461–5
Tillich P 1954 Love, power and justice. Oxford University Press
Townsend P, Davidson N 1982 Inequalities in health: The Black Report. Penguin Books, Harmondsworth

United Nations Organisation, 1948 Universal Declaration of Human Rights. UNO New York. Also reproduced in: Campbell A V 1978 Medicine health and justice. Churchill Livingstone, Edinburgh

Veatch R 1981 A theory of medical ethics. Basic Books, New York

White R 1970 Social change and the development of nursing. Kimpton, London

Whitehead M 1987 The health divide. Health Education Council, London

WHO 1978 Primary health care. Report of international conference held at Alma Ata, USSR. World Health Organisation, Geneva

WHO 1981 Regional programme in health education and life-styles (31st Session of Regional Committee for Europe), EUR/RC31/10. World Health Organisation, Copenhagen

WHO 1979 Primary health care in Europe. Euro Reports on Studies No 14. World Health Organisation, Copenhagen

5

What are the key moral issues in health care?

The expectations of most nurses, at least judging from the nursing press and experience of discussion with student nurses, is that nursing ethics has to do with the big dilemmas such as abortion, euthanasia, truth-telling, compulsory psychiatric treatment. This is understandable, for when these problems arise in the direct nurse–patient relationship they focus directly on the tensions between people's personal feelings, moral beliefs and professional responsibilities. These issues are important and cannot be avoided, but it should perhaps be emphasised that as a professional carer, paid to provide care, the nurse also has wider social responsibilities in a public role as a kind of public servant, official or health service employee. The moral problems and dilemmas which arise in the exercise of the public office of 'nurse' are no less important and, in senior posts, often involve much heavier responsibility. The ethical issues here arise in the wider responsibilities of nurses to groups of patients, relationships with colleagues and accountability to employers and the general public. These areas of responsibility are often regarded as more 'political' but are really continuous with the direct and intimate problems of patient care. Perhaps by regarding them as political we implicitly recognise that they raise questions at the macro level about the basis of our moral beliefs and ideological commitments, whereas the familiar dilemmas relate to the micro level, that is, to specific problems or dilemmas raised by conflicts *within* our accepted systems of beliefs (Campbell 1985, White 1985).

5.1 Health and disease as personal and social values

We cannot avoid making moral choices or debating matters of moral principle in health care since the whole question of our health — as individuals, in family life, in our work and in society — is not a matter of indifference to us. We all desire good health and seek to avoid pain and injury, disease and death. The illness or handicap of a parent or one family member can affect the well-being of all the others. Work-related accidents or absenteeism caused by illness affects the productivity of organisations and industry, often more seriously than strikes. The cost of caring for the sick, injured, mentally disordered, severely handicapped, senile and dying is a burden on any society — a burden first of all in human terms on those in families who bear the brunt of most of the anxiety and direct care, and a burden, too, on the state in providing primary care and hospital services, and on the professional staff who are paid to care (Wilson 1976).

'Health' and 'disease' are terms with several meanings — scientific and medical meanings, and more popular meanings that relate to ideal states of personal and social well-being or states of personal and social disorder we wish to avoid. Even in physiology and pathology 'health' and 'disease' are *normative terms*, that is, they describe the state of an organism as approaching ideal or optimum functioning or varying degrees of malfunctioning or dysfunction — within a continuum where health is at one pole and disease at the other. At a more personal level, we do not have to be 'health freaks' in order to want to be healthy, because most of the things we do, most of the things that give us pleasure, are more fun, more enjoyable when we are fit and healthy than if we are unfit, ill or injured. Good health is something we value. It is an ideal we strive to realise for ourselves (and perhaps for others). So, too, disease is an evil we try to avoid or prevent, or failing both, to cure. The World Health Organisation recognised that health and disease are personal and social values and not simply medical labels in the famous definition: 'Health is complete physical, mental and social well-being and not just the absence of disease, or infirmity' (WHO 1947).

In attempting to define health we raise fundamental ethical, political and even religious questions about values and life-choices, even before we get into specific questions about the personal and moral responsibilities of nurses and other health-professionals in paid service to others, or wider philosophical debate about the nature of health services and the best systems for effective and efficient delivery of health care (Seedhouse 1986).

In making decisions about our *personal health*, we have to make both practical and moral choices about our behaviour and lifestyle if we are to live healthy lives and avoid accidents, injury, disease or premature death. Alternatively, while we may tend to regard attempted suicide as a sign of mental disorder in an individual, the decision to end one's life prematurely either by direct suicide or by taking risks that may result in death, is also a moral choice. However, we do not exist in splendid isolation and our lives touch and inter-lock with those of others in many different ways — in family life, in our friendships and love affairs, in our work and recreation. Just as an attempted or actual suicide can cause intense pain and grief to many other people, so too in a less dramatic way illness, injury or personal distress can and does affect other people.

Society is and has to be interested in the health and well-being of its members. First because we are part of one another, second because the whole human family may suffer if we are unable to make or are prevented from making our own contribution to society, and third because of the additional burden and cost of care and treatment that may result.

Public health education and public health measures such as immunisation, screening, the imposition of quarantines and travel restrictions, compulsory notification of diseases, and general controls on sanitary supply of food, water and sewerage/waste disposal and environmental controls on housing, provision of public amenities and health services are all undertaken by the state in order to prevent disease and to promote the health of society.

There is a potential conflict right here at the beginning between personal liberty to do what we want in pursuing the lifestyle of our choice, and the well-intentioned but often officious and interfering attempts of family, friends, school and health professionals, mass media and political agencies to change or redirect health behaviour. These issues involve basic ethical questions about personal rights and social responsibility and the wider good of society and so have general relevance to the ethics of health care, but also in a more particular way often to nursing ethics. Nurses are often involved in conflicts between what they preach and what they practise. As front-line health educators with a professional responsibility to prevent disease as well as to care for and treat those who are ill, nurses have to face the conflicts between their own health behaviour (e.g. with regard to smoking, drug or alcohol abuse, diet, fitness, responsible sex) and what they are advising their patients or clients to do. The issues are not only about the expectations relating to the nurse or health professional as a role model, but also about their function as educators or agents of social control.

For example, health education can be presented in such a way as to encourage us to know more about healthy living, to make informed choices and to take responsibility for our own health and choice of lifestyle. Alternatively, health propaganda may seek to redirect our behaviour, either by persuasion, or by subtle or not so subtle legal coercion. Aggressive promotion of healthy lifestyles by state agencies has to be justified by a kind of healthist ideology, whereas traditional preventive medicine simply sought to prevent disease. This is not necessarily to be condemned, rather we should understand what kind of values are being promoted and be willing to examine and challenge these. On the one hand, millions of pounds are spent annually by the tobacco, alcohol and junk food industries on advertising and sponsorship to promote the sale of products that are damaging to health. On the other hand, we increasingly see the alliance of state propaganda with our commercial interests in the marketing of health (sports equipment and clothing, public spectaculars and mass participation in spectator sports). The public fashion for jogging, health foods, diet and fitness is not just a product of individual people's desire to be fit and healthy. It is the result of many factors including personal interest, and raised awareness of health as an issue in people's lives, but also of an orchestrated attempt of political and commercially controlled media advertising to 'market' health as an ideology and to change people's health behaviour and lifestyles accordingly (Ewles & Simnett 1985).

When Health For All by the Year 2000 was adopted at the Alma-Ata International Conference of the World Health Organisation in 1978 as a policy objective (WHO 1978), this was dismissed by many cynics as wildly optimistic, impractical and unattainable. However, by setting such a goal, the World Health Organisation has encouraged UN member states to formulate specific attainable objectives and action plans to achieve this target. As a result, member states have adopted and begun to implement programmes of health promotion, disease prevention and reorientation of resources to primary care that may well change the face of health care in the next century (WHO 1981). This has come about, and is coming about, through attention to the ethical and political implications of good health as something of personal and social value. If we start by recognising that 'health' and 'disease' are value terms, then we will be obliged to see that the discussion of moral problems and responsibilities around direct patient care fall within the broader commitments we make as individuals, professionals and members of society to achieve good health. These may include individual and pressure-group activity either to promote good health for all and to encourage people to help themselves to health, or to raise public awareness and mobilise public support for fiscal, legal and other controls on the advertising and marketing of products which will damage our health.

5.2 The 'big dilemmas' of nursing ethics

It is not the broader issues of public and community health that nurses think of first when the ethics of health care is raised. Although the issues around health education are increasingly important, the dilemmas of treatment and those related to the provision of therapeutic services tend to have greater prominence.

The reasons for this are complex and various, for example: most health professionals are trained within the crisis-oriented treatment services rather than in prevention; so-called health services are in practice more concerned with the treatment of disease; and, indeed, with the bulk of the money and resources going into research and treatment in the therapeutic services, the power and prestige tend to be concentrated there (HMSO 1978). Whether or not diagnostic and treatment services or public health measures are more effective in improving the health of society (McKeown 1979), the image of hi-technology medicine and intensive care nursing is more attractive and the focus on individual patients and their problems has more human appeal. Similarly, although the majority of nurses will be employed in long-term care of the chronic sick, the mentally ill and the elderly, it is midwifery, paediatric nursing, acute medical and surgical and terminal care nursing which enjoy higher prestige and glamour. This influences our perception of what issues are ethically most important.

The standard examples of big dilemmas in medical ethics given in recent books on ethics for health professionals, whether written for doctors, nurses or paramedics, tend to be the same, regardless of the profound differences between the roles and responsibilities of each profession. While there may be important things to be learned for all health professionals from the consideration of general topics — such as abortion or euthanasia, truth-telling or confidentiality, compulsory psychiatric treatment or *in vitro* fertilisation, dilemmas of resource allocation or management accountability — nevertheless, the specific issues of importance to nurses may be very different from those aspects of the topics of importance to doctors or other professional staff.

The issues common to all health professionals relate to the way *power* (or control) *is exercised* over people, *or power shared* with people — whether people seek their help voluntarily or are committed into their care by relatives or other authorities. While the division of responsibility and/or authority may differ in the ward or in the primary care team; and while many of the frustrations of nurses may focus on the fact that they often have responsibility without executive authority, it would be a mistake to overlook the very real and proper responsibilities of nurses as distinct from doctors.

The issues about which nurses probably bother most tend to be those which relate directly to their spheres of personal responsibility in either direct patient care or management roles, rather than the more general and intractable issues where they feel they can personally do very little or which are beyond their control. Issues around communication with patients (truth-telling and confidentiality) and conflicts with doctors, other carers and relatives over patient care, tend to predominate. Nurses may well have an intellectual interest in a wide range of current moral issues in health care, and some nurses may have particular reasons to object to assisting with abortions or be worried by requests from patients for euthanasia, but in practice they can also distance themselves from a lot of issues as not being their responsibility but the doctor's.

In many cases nurses may feel relatively powerless in so far as others in more powerful positions (e.g. doctors or the competent legal authorities) take decisions which affect the admission or discharge of patients or the form of treatment which they are to receive. In this sense nurses are not in control and inherit responsibilities which flow from decisions others have taken for them and which they may feel powerless to change or influence. Most of the classic big dilemmas are problems in law or medical ethics before they become problems for nurses. However, this is not to say that these problems and dilemmas do not present in a different way in nursing, or that nurses do not have unique and distinctive responsibilities, or that nursing ethics does not have a unique contribution to make to the debate about these issues. In fact if nurses were to focus their concern and frustration on their perceived powerlessness relative to doctors and to see nursing ethics only as a kind of commentary on or vicarious participation in medical ethics, then it would be hardly worth pursuing.

In reality, nurses do have considerable power over patients. The way they decide on the allocation of staff time and ward or community resources can directly influence both the quantity and quality of care given to patients. They can influence the patient both directly and indirectly by the way they change or manipulate the patient's environment. They can influence both directly and indirectly the decisions of doctors, paramedics and other carers, about the appropriateness or inappropriateness of treatment, levels of pain control, compulsory detention in hospital or discharge, by the nature and quality of their observations regarding the patient's physical, emotional and psychological state. They can influence management about necessary organisational and institutional change, or campaign for more resources, and in general have a responsibility to maintain general standards of patient care. While individual nurses may have reason to object to carrying out doctor's orders, whether in administering drugs with potentially fatal side-effects, assisting with abortions, offering euthanasia or administering ECT (electro-convulsive therapy) — the real focus of concern in nursing ethics should be on those areas where nurses have specific responsibility which are different from those of other health professionals or social workers. These areas which relate to such matters as the organisation of the patient's day, skilled attention to the patient's physical, psychological and emotional needs, humanisation of the environment and counteracting institutionalisation and dependency are often overlooked while more attention is given to the big dilemmas of medical ethics.

5.3 The 'medicalisation of life' and the 'big dilemmas'

One way of looking at the big dilemmas of direct patient care, which we listed above, is to see them as having become issues of importance in medicine and nursing through a process which Illich has called 'the medicalisation of life' (Illich 1977). According to his analysis, doctors and other health professionals have effectively become the priests of modern society, presiding over and controlling all the crucial 'rites of passage' from birth to death. The treatment of disease, injury and mental disorder, and concern with health promotion, have come to embrace the whole of life and all its stages.

Health professionals are directly involved in giving treatment for infertility or advice on fertility control; antenatal preparation or termination of pregnancy; assistance with childbirth and supervision of post-natal care and screening for

abnormalities; monitoring of physical and psychological
child-development; medical and psychiatric treatment of the
disorders of adolescence; advice and treatment of nutritional
disorders, drug dependency, sexual and marital problems;
prescription of rest, exercise or recreation; supervision,
custodial care and treatment of the mentally disordered,
severely mentally handicapped and senile: and finally orches-
tration of the predeath counselling, terminal care and post-
death follow-up of the bereaved.

The 'medicalisation' of life has meant that health
professionals have inherited some of the power and control
over matters of life and death which in more traditional
society have been the domain of priests and religious healers.
Faith in religion and in divine judgement or providential care
has yielded to a large degree to faith in secular science and
the 'miracles' of modern medicine. As health professionals
have come to supervise and control the 'rites of passage'
relating to our key life-events, so they have acquired
awesome, even god-like, responsibility for making life-and-
death decisions.

Illich's book (Illich 1977) is a critique of the dominance
which doctors have come to exercise over our lives and the
temptations they face to 'play God'. Nurses often use his
arguments to reinforce many of their criticisms of the arrogance and assumed moral superiority of doctors. However,
the implications of Illich's analysis go much further and relate
to the role of nurses too — whether in the traditional role of
'doctor's handmaidens' or as modern self-consciously independent health professionals with distinctive roles and
responsibilities of their own. In both cases nurses are part of
the process and the system which has resulted in this medicalisation of life, with its corresponding removal from ordinary people of the power of decision and responsibility for
their own lives. It is arguable, too, that while the power of
priests and religious healers was limited by acknowledgement
of a transcendent divine power and authority, secular health
care is subject to no such limitations.

In the first instance, then, the big dilemmas such as abortion, secrecy and truth-telling, fertility control/treatment of
infertility, compulsory psychiatric treatment and euthanasia or
the right to die are a direct consequence and inheritance of

this power and responsibility associated with the medicalisation of life. Obviously, we need to look at the specific issues
raised by each of these big dilemmas, but it may be useful to
bear in mind this general historical analysis and be prepared
to consider its broader implications too.

5.4 Individual 'health careers' and professional control

A complementary type of analysis, based on developmental
psychology, has come up with the concept of a 'health career'
(Baric 1974, Dorn & Nortoft 1982). As we grow from infancy
through childhood to maturity and decline into old age and
die, our life passes through a series of ups and downs.

On the one hand, the whole of our life career could be
represented by a parabolic curve starting with conception,
rising to the peak of our physical and mental development
and curving down to meet the horizontal axis again at death.
Along that line, our progress is not necessarily smooth; it has
its 'ups' when we are healthy and things are going well for
us, and its 'downs' when we are sick, suffer injury or external
factors limit and arrest our development. As we get better, or
get over a crisis in our lives, so we regain some of the lost
ground and our development continues. As we get past
middle age or suffer severe illness or disabling injury, so our
capacity for recovery becomes more limited and our general
condition may decline, until we finally succumb to the disin-
tegrating effect of disease, injury and the wear-and-tear of old
age, and die. Some people may live a long time with a very
steady rhythm, other people's lives may be marked by
numerous crises, others may be cut short tragically by
sudden, accidental or violent death. It is possible to examine
the medicalisation of life across the whole span of an individual's health career, but it is also illuminating to apply it to
the specific analysis of smaller sections of people's lives or
individual episodes of illness, injury or mental disorder.

If we map the passage of an individual from a state of relative health and independence through some health crisis
where they become relatively or completely dependent on
help from others, and then recover and return gradually to
something like their former state of health and independence, this process can be illustrated on a simple graph by an

inverted parabolic curve. On such a graph the horizontal axis would represent the continuous time-line and on the vertical axis we could represent various degrees of autonomy above the line and various degrees of dependency below the line.

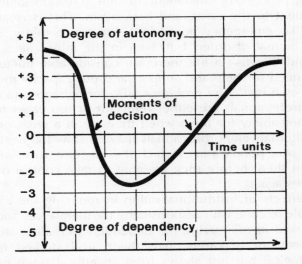

When a healthy person who is, say, lucid, mobile, continent and independent experiences some health crisis (through injury, disease or environmental insult) they may rapidly decline into a state of relative or deep dependency on others, from which they have to be assisted to recover. The process of assisting people to get back 'on to their feet' we call rehabilitation. The deeper the downward curve the more total will be the carer's *responsibility* for the person entrusted into their care, but as they are assisted to recovery, or recover spontaneously, then the carer has to assist them back to recovery and independence, not to keep them in a state of perpetual dependence.

There are two points of *crisis* (moments of decision, from Greek *krino*, to judge or decide) in this process: first, when the individual hands over responsibility to the carer, or is handed over to them; and second, when responsibility is handed back to the patient or client. The crossing of the horizontal axis by the downward and upward movement of the line illustrating this episode in the individual's health career, makes these crisis-points on the parabolic curve, at the boundary-line between autonomy and dependency.

What is important about this model for illustrating a person's health career is that it emphasises that there is a dynamic process, or movement, or shift in responsibility from the patient to the carer, and back again. This is clearest in cases like emergency admissions for major injury, or for severe mental disorder, but even in the minor illnesses or 'ups' and 'downs' in life there are considerable fluctuations in our need for help and support and our capacity to 'stand on our own feet'. The problems arise for patients and clients when professionals are either reluctant or too eager to take on responsibility for them when they are in a crisis or need help. Alternatively, professionals may be slow to give up the control over people's lives which they acquire, or too readily abandon them before they are able to take control of their own lives again.

The effects of institutionalisation in reducing the capacity of people to cope with responsibility for themselves and their health, and in reinforcing the dependency-creating attitudes and behaviour of carers, have been well studied from a psychological but not always from an ethical point of view (Goffman 1961). This particularly applies to the often unwanted moral responsibilities which carers inherit as a result of taking on people in need. Where the health crisis requires emergency treatment, the pressures on the carer to take urgent life-and-death decisions may be considerable. They may well find it emotionally costly and physically exhausting, may resent being left 'carrying the can', and may feel exaggerated guilt if things go wrong.

Ethical codes in the caring professions have mainly focused on the responsibility the carer accepts for the client, few have stressed the importance of the commitment the carer must make to return control to the client as soon as he is again capable of being independent. None of the existing medical codes stresses this moral duty in the rehabilitation of patients, but significantly both the International Council of Nurses and the Royal College of Nursing seem to say that the primary duty of the nurse is to work to restore autonomy to the individual who has lost it as a result of illness, injury or mental disorder. These statements emphasise a value funda-

mental to nursing ethics which appears to arise out of reflection on the distinctive nature of nursing care.

5.5 Ethical analysis of the 'big dilemmas'

One of the consequences of the medicalisation of life is not
only that health professionals have acquired increased
responsibility for the care of people from birth to death,
along with greater power and control over their lives, but they
have also acquired moral responsibility for decisions in areas
ranging from promotion of fertility to termination of pregnancy, organ transplants and the artificial prolongation of life
by mechanical aids to assisting patients to a good death
(euthanasia, from Greek *eu*, good, and *thanatos*, death).
Some carers 'enjoy' the power and responsibility involved,
others find it a painful burden, but no one can remain indifferent. The big dilemmas tend to focus on some of the key
issues and must be addressed, particularly if we are to clarify
the different roles and responsibilities of doctors, nurses and
other carers in dealing with these problem situations.

It is difficult to restrict the list of big dilemmas for
discussion but the following seem to be a perennial source
of concern: abortion and euthanasia; truth-telling and confidentiality; compulsory psychiatric treatment; and problems
relating to management accountability and reconciling the
conflicting demands of different patients with limited
resources. Part of the problem with these issues is that they
each raise important questions of general principle and we
therefore tend to discuss them in general terms or in the
abstract. This does not help very much when we are
confronted with urgent problems of particular people in their
specific circumstances and situation of crisis demanding our
help. Furthermore, in real life there will usually be several
parties with different interests and possible conflicting points
of view about what their rights and responsibilities are.

Abortion and euthanasia: The right to life and the right to die

From the dawn of time women have sought assistance to
terminate unwanted pregnancies, whether or not this has

been permitted by law or morality. If help has been refused or unavailable, women have attempted by an infinite variety of means to effect an abortion themselves or have resorted to infanticide. Some societies have tolerated abortion, but it has generally been prohibited and those seeking to procure or assisting with abortions have been severely punished. In a sense it is only with liberal legislation which has decrimina- lised abortion that the issue has, strictly speaking, become a matter of clinical and moral responsibility for nurses. Of course, nurses have had to grapple with the problem before the Abortion Act in Britain, for example, and nurses will have had views on the morality or immorality of abortion before 1967, but it is only since that time that nurses as nurses in Britain, and particularly in the National Health Service, have had to face the issues as a direct challenge to nursing ethics. For the nurse, or midwife specifically, it might be argued that there is an immediate and apparent contradiction between the responsibility to protect, nurture and save life, and the responsibility for the wider care of the woman for whom an unwanted pregnancy is a personal disaster.

The issue of *abortion* is usually debated from the pro-life point of view in terms of the sanctity of life or the rights of the unborn child. From the point of view of those that favour further liberalisation of the law and moral attitudes on abor- tion, the issue is about women's rights and and in particular their right to control their own fertility including recourse to termination of pregnancy. Relatives and wider society tend to enter the debate in an attempt either to protect the unborn child or to defend the woman. Here the issues tend to be raised in wider terms of justice and the common good. The health professionals often tend to get left out of the debate, except where they are called in as expert witnesses, but in reality they are often left playing 'piggy in the middle'. The duty to care for both mother and child leaves them in an impossible situation, e.g. where they have to choose between the life of the one or the other. The conflicting demands of such a situation cannot be resolved by carers consulting their consciences about which individual (mother or baby) they owe a greater duty of care. Other considerations of personal rights and justice have to be taken into account, and the tension between these conflicting values in real life is what make these problems so painful and face us with apparently unsolvable dilemmas.

The sanctity of life argument that so easily leads on to claims that abortion is murder, raises both fundamental issues and insuperable problems in ethics. If all life is sacred, where do you draw the line? With the newborn, the fetus, the conceptus, the ovum or individual sperm . . . or where? Is it only human life that is sacred or is it animal and vegetable life as well? If we say human life, when does life become human in the continuum between individual cell and adult person? Attempts to legislate that *human life* begins at conception, or that the fetus acquires legal and moral rights at quickening (when ensoulment was supposed to take place), or at 28 weeks gestation, or only at birth, or at puberty, or at age 21 years, do not solve the fundamental problem of what is meant by a person with rights or how to define membership of the moral community.

Dogmatic definitions simply foreclose rational debate and exploration of these complex questions to which fundamentally different answers have been given in different societies and cultures. In Hinduism, where all living things are regarded as sacred — and strict vegans would not kill any animal or eat animal products — the moral community is so broad as to include all living things as having rights. At the other extreme, the Nazis sought to restrict the moral community to pure Aryans, and other 'lesser' races were denied fundamental moral rights or even the protection of the law. In Western culture we tend to have regarded only human beings as having moral rights or qualifying as members of the moral community and have extended protection to animals on the grounds that cruelty or abuse of animals is inhuman, not that animals as such have rights. The animal liberation movements have sought to challenge this view. Furthermore, within our own culture we have been very confused about whether all human beings — including women and children — slaves, and the mentally and physically handicapped should enjoy full human rights. The present legal debate about *in vitro* fertilisation is bedevilled by confusion about where we draw the line in experiments with embryos, because the law on the one hand acknowledges the right of the unborn child to inherit property or to recover damages for injury suffered *in utero*, but on the other hand abrogates the unborn child's right to life in permitting abortion, under specific conditions.

This analysis is not meant to decide the abortion issue one way or the other, but rather to raise a fundamental series of questions in ethics. What do we mean by a 'person'? What do we mean by respect for personal dignity and rights? What do we mean by membership of the moral community? Who qualifies for membership? What rights and responsibilities does membership entail?

Perhaps ironically those who campaign for women's rights and the right to termination of pregnancy fail to recognise that the very claims which they make rest upon assumptions about respect for persons as bearers of rights and members of the moral community which are raised by debate about the moral and legal status of pre-natal life. Whether women should enjoy equal rights with men, should be protected from sexual domination or exploitation by men, should be given equal opportunities for care and treatment within health services (which institutionalise the values of male-dominated society), are all issues which relate back fundamentally to the principle of respect for persons and how we define the rights and responsibilities of members of the moral community (Campbell 1972, Rumbold 1986).

Issues round euthanasia and compulsory psychiatric treatment relate to extremes in the balance of power between carer and client and the tensions which such situations generate between the requirements of the duty-to-care — to protect the vulnerable and incompetent — on the one hand; and respect for the autonomy and personal rights of the client on the other hand.

Euthanasia is a term used rather loosely. Sometimes it is used to cover the situation where a carer of their own initiative assists the patient to a good death — whether that involves withholding treatment (passive euthanasia), or administering a drug or treatment which hastens death (active euthanasia). In either situation the carer would probably justify this action in terms of an extension of their duty to care — to prevent unnecessary suffering, for example. However, the term 'euthanasia' is also used where the patient requests assistance to put an end to their suffering, or has requested in advance (perhaps in a sworn statement) that they do not wish their lives artificially prolonged if their condition is terminal. This kind of 'voluntary euthanasia' involves the patient or client insisting on respect of their personal wishes and claiming the 'right' to die, or at least to be consulted about the scope and limits of what we euphemistically call 'terminal care'.

Where the carer feels compelled to act to put an end to the hopeless suffering of a patient, there is an inevitable clash between the values and principles which protect the integrity of individuals and their right to life (including the prohibition of murder or assisted suicide), and the overwhelming desire of the carer to see someone who is struggling in painful death put out of their misery. Alternatively, the carer may feel pressurised by the patient who demands respect for their 'right' to die. The nurse may feel that nursing care is about sustaining life, not about assisting patients to kill themselves or to hasten their death. Nurses generally feel that no patient has any genuine right to demand that the nurse terminate his life.

The Voluntary Euthanasia Society has long campaigned for the legalisation of voluntary euthanasia, but there seemed to be insuperable legal obstacles as long as attempted suicide was illegal. When the Suicide Act of 1961 was passed, suicide and attempted suicide ceased to be criminal acts in England (they had never been so regarded in Scotland). Supporters of the Voluntary Euthanasia Society claimed a moral victory and argued that the Suicide Act created a legal 'right to die'. This argument was based on a misunderstanding of the extent of the Act as an 'enabling' Act. What the legislation did was to decriminalise suicide and attempted suicide; it conceded that people may be *allowed the liberty* to take their own lives without suffering the penalties of the criminal law. But did the Act create a positive legal *right* to die?

Generally speaking, moral and legal rights are justified claims that entitle us to demand that other people act or desist from acting in certain ways — that is, our 'rights' impose either positive or negative duties on others. Moral rights have only the strength which existing social consensus and convention give them, and impose only moral obligations on others, whereas legal rights may be enforceable through the courts.

In the strong sense, the Suicide Act does not create a *right to die* which is legally enforceable, that is, by imposing on anyone else a legal duty to assist one to die, or not to prevent one taking one's own life. In fact the Homicide Act of 1957 specifically precludes the former by making assisted suicide a form of criminal homicide, and various provisions of the Mental Health Act make it possible for both health professionals and lay people to take action to have persons detained in hospital compulsorily if they are considered a serious suicide risk. In the weaker sense, of the individual being allowed the *liberty* in law to attempt suicide, it may be argued that in cases of patients dying in extreme pain or undignified circumstances others may feel an obligation to assist them to an easy or good death. However, neither law nor public morality concedes that anyone has a right to demand the assistance of another person to terminate their life. In practice, some nurses (or doctors) may feel moved to stop treatment or life support, or may actively intervene to terminate the life of someone in extreme suffering by the administration of drugs or by other means. However, such action would be illegal, whatever the circumstances, and in most cases would not be morally sanctioned either because carers are expected to sustain life not end it, and most societies have in fact moral principles forbidding suicide except in the most extreme circumstances (Thompson 1976).

The provisions of the law and the constraints of public morality may or may not suffice to help the nurse in a particular case to decide whether to refuse the desperate request from a patient for deliverance from a living death. However, the introduction of legislation permitting voluntary euthanasia would not resolve the dilemmas for nurses or doctors either, as no law could impose on them the duty to perform euthanasia against their will or conscience, nor remove the painful tension between the duty to care and respect for the dignity of the suffering patient. Neither could such legislation adequately prevent the misuse of euthanasia by unscrupulous individuals who might benefit from another's death. That is why we seem stuck with Arthur

Clough's ironic wisdom: 'Thou shalt not kill, but needst not strive officiously to keep alive' (Mulhauser 1974).

This is not to make light of the painful issues faced by carers and their patients in situations of terminal illness. In fact, another irony which emerges in terminal care is that if staff work to support and respect the autonomy of dying patients, to discuss the implications of their imminent death with them, to support them through the anticipatory grief and distress, to consult them and respect their wishes on how, when and where they are to die, then good terminal care, which was supposed to be an alternative to voluntary euthanasia, actually approximates to it. If terminal care is not 'assisting patients to a good death', what is it? The pain and the dilemmas do not go away, although each case may be sensitively handled in a quite different way. No universal prescriptions are possible or would be appropriate (Thompson 1984a).

Dilemmas of truth-telling and confidentiality: Information-sharing and information-control

Dilemmas of truth-telling and confidentiality arise because of apparent or actual conflicts between the patient's rights and the carer's duty to care. The classic situation of whether and when to tell the dying patients that their condition is terminal illustrates the tension between two opposing moral concerns: first, respect for the patients' autonomy and right to know on the one hand, and, second, the feeling of the carer that she should protect the patients from news which may shock and distress them, perhaps causing them to give up in despair. The situation in practice may be complicated by the intervention of relatives demanding to know or forbidding communication with the dying, by the hope or anxiety that the fatal diagnosis might be wrong, by the various parties involved not wishing to acknowledge failure or to relinquish control or simply to protect themselves from the emotional burden of the dying patient's grief. It is difficult to discuss these subtle problems of communication with the dying, which require great sensitivity, trust and confidence in the relationships of carers, patients and relatives. They are not susceptible to universal prescriptions and the predicament of nurses may be that in practice they are prevented by 'doctor's orders' from doing what they believe to be the best in the circumstances. However, what makes these issues perennial dilemmas is that they bring opposing rights and duties into painful conflict. Whether priority will be given to the patient's right to know or to the professional's duty to protect the vulnerability of the dying patient cannot be decided by mere appeal to principle but has to be worked out in the complexity of each unique situation, in the way that seems most caring and responsible at the time (Thompson 1984a).

Respect for the patient's secrets, their right to privacy, is again complicated by the often overriding duty to care and to do what is in the best interests of the patient. This may involve the carer in passing on confidential information to another professional in the hope that it will assist in the better care of their confidant. Ideally the carer has a duty to seek the consent of their confidant before sharing their secrets, but if it it not possible to get it, then the dilemma arises: which is to take precedence — the patient's right to privacy or the professional's duty to provide the best possible care for the patient? Dilemmas of confidentiality do not arise out of careless disclosures of patients' secrets, but rather when the responsibilities of nurses to their patients, for example, come into conflict with the requirements of team management of patient care or in sharing information with relatives.

Possession of sensitive confidential information about clients or patients is often both a burden and responsibility of carers, but it also gives them a special relationship with those in their care and subtle power over them. Carers are often inclined jealously to guard this private information and are reluctant to share it with colleagues because it means compromising the special relationship they have with 'their' patients/clients. Within the changing situation of the carer/client relationship, as the client enters a crisis and becomes increasingly dependent so the carer acquires greater power and control over the life of the client. Part of this control consists in management of the flow of information to the client, from the client and about the client. Giving or withholding information is a powerful way of encouraging co-operation or compliance and maintaining control in the caring relationship. Because knowledge is power and to be kept in ignorance is to be kept in a state of dependence, the manner in which the information and confidences are shared is a sensitive indicator of whether professional attitudes are creating dependency or whether they are used to assist the client towards autonomy, to take control of their own lives again (Thompson 1979).

Compulsory psychiatric treatment: For whose benefit?

The dilemmas of confidentiality and truth-telling, as well as general conflicts between protective beneficence and respect for a person's rights arise in the most acute form where the patient or client has become incompetent. Society may require that the individual who is mentally disordered or becoming senile is taken into hospital against his will, and even subjected to compulsory treatment. Deciding whether an individual should be compulsorily detained in hospital may be relatively easy in cases of severe dementia or florid mental illness, but the vast majority of psychiatric cases are not so clear-cut. The legal requirement that the individual must be a danger to themselves or others is extremely difficult to determine in practice. To avoid public criticism or legal action for negligence, caring staff may tend to err on the side of caution and thus compromise the rights of individuals when the degree of danger would be virtually impossible to assess.

Furthermore, the individual who is admitted in a severely disturbed state may recover without treatment, or may have periods of reasonable normality and periods where they are clearly incompetent. Whether the system is sensitive enough to respond to these changes in the moral status of the detained patient and to respect their right to information or to be consulted about their treatment, may be doubted. The peculiar disabling effect of mental disorders, in affecting the patient's competence to exercise responsibility and to control or direct their lives, makes it peculiarly difficult to decide at what stage in the rehabilitation process it is appropriate for the carer to relinquish control. Conservative and defensive practice on the part of carers can thus encourage chronic dependency.

There are several peculiar features of the medical treatment of mental illness which create moral difficulties or dilemmas for nurses. These problems arise because of ambiguities in the diagnosis, treatment and rehabilitation of people with mental illness (including senile dementia and severe mental handicap). These ambiguities are to be found: in the moral/legal status of the patient; in the definition and diagnosis of 'mental illness'; in the variety of activities which count as 'treatment'; in the definition of which patients are the carer's responsibility.

The ambiguous moral/legal status of someone suffering from a mental disorder is reflected in the fact that health professionals have unique legal powers to detain and treat patients who are mentally ill. The central paradox of psychiatry is that a person may have to be deprived of their liberty and treated against their will in the hope that this will make it possible to restore their autonomy and enable them to take control of their lives again. To justify the extraordinary legal powers taken by professionals against mentally disordered individuals, the law requires proof that the person is a danger to others or at risk to themselves. In these terms the professionals' legally reinforced duty to care supposedly rests on the moral demands of protective beneficence (in preventing others from harm and defending the common good). To protect the rights of the patient, various legal safeguards and rights of appeal tend to be built into mental health legislation and there is recourse to the courts or mental health tribunals for independent review of patients and their care. But serious questions may be asked about whose good the system serves, whether the mentally ill (with a few exceptions) are really a danger to others, and whether legal action is justified to restrain suicidal patients who are allegedly ill if attempted suicide is not a course for 'normal' people.

The notorious imprecision of definitions of mental illness, and even serious disagreement whether mental illness exists (as distinct from physiological disorders, or emotional distress and problems of living), makes it at least questionable whether individuals who are diagnosed as suffering from some kind of 'mental' disorder should be singled out for special legal sanctions, deprivation of liberty and the denial of their fundamental rights — for example, the right to informed and voluntary consent to treatment, the right to privacy and confidentiality (compromised in group therapy and team management), the right to refuse treatment and discharge themselves from hospital. The dubious benefits of a psychiatric diagnosis (asylum, access to care and treatment, relief from the burden of family or work responsibility) have to be counterbalanced against the disabling and stigmatising effect of being labelled mentally ill.

In psychiatry, the contract to participate in prescribed treatment is wider and more inclusive than perhaps any other area of medicine — ranging from mere asylum, individual and group psychotherapy, and an enormous range of occupational therapies (art, music, dance, employment), physiotherapy and behaviour therapy, to chemotherapy, ECT and psychosurgery. It is by no means clear to the average patient, or nurse for that matter, what the scope or limits of 'treatment' in the case of any given patient will include. There is a risk that health professionals will arrogate to themselves the right to decide 'what are in the best interests of the patient' without consulting the patient or relative. For the compulsorily detained patient, co-operation and compliance can be elicited by the mere hint of the extension of compulsory powers or their reimposition. Nurses are intimately involved in the whole complex of relationships which operate and sustain these systems in psychiatric and psychogeriatric institutions.

Community psychiatry or the investigation of the family background of a psychiatric patient raises serious questions for the nurse in dealing with the family. Who is the patient? Who are included within the scope of the responsibility of the community psychiatric nurse? Has the nurse the right to intervene in the family life of the patient? To draw other family members into the therapeutic net? Again, the situation is without parallel (except perhaps in contact tracing in venereal disease). Do health professionals have a right to seek out undisclosed pathology, or undeclared patients who have not recognised that they have a problem? Because the legal powers taken in psychiatry are extraordinary, they raise all sorts of questions about the scope and limits of professional responsibility and the rights and status of patients/family (Thompson 1984b).

Management accountability and dilemmas in allocation of resources

All the examples discussed tend to occur within one-to-one relationships in patient care, where the primary tension is between the professional's duty to care and protect the patient, and the demand that the carer respects the dignity and rights of the patient/client as a person. There is a whole class of other dilemmas which arise in the relationships between carers and two or more clients. While we will discuss other examples of these one-to-many dilemmas, the ones which are raised most frequently in discussion are on the borderline between problems of direct patient care and management. Such cases might be illustrated when there are two candidates for intensive care or kidney dialysis and facilities for the treatment of only one. Alternatively, the case may be about the possible diversion of resources from expensive treatment of a few patients to larger groups of chronic patients, say geriatric patients. Leaving aside technical clinical considerations which would be relevant, and might in some cases help to decide the issues, the moral question is fundamentally about justice. It concerns the right of everyone to equal access to appropriate care and treatment, particularly in a system of health care to which all contribute by taxation directly or indirectly. The claims of certain individuals, either because they are wealthier, more powerful or just more attractive human beings, have to be balanced against the common good. The priorities determined by professionals on their own criteria for giving certain clients preference over others because 'in need of greater care' may also have to be challenged or questioned in the name of justice, if others suffer neglect as a result (Boyd 1979).

The dilemmas of responsibility and accountability in nurse management roles are not restricted to dilemmas in the allocation of limited resources or reconciling conflicting needs of different patients. There are some prosaic problems about the management and deployment of staff, the management of time and resources in the routine care of large groups of patients, and the choices which have to be made between the balance of time spent on patient care and/or patient education, teaching or research and evaluation.

All these management roles are inherently political — political in the sense that they involve balancing interests and powers within the institution, negotiating with higher authority outwith the institution about policy, staffing, wages, resources, and using collective action through professional or union organisations to seek better working conditions for nurses and to maintain or achieve better standards of patient care. Issues of the rights of patients versus the rights of nurses, of the duties of nurses and the duties of patients, of justice in the sense of non-discrimination against individuals, and equality of opportunity and outcome for groups, of the duty to care for vulnerable patients, and the duty to care for staff all involve the same fundamental moral principles. However, different tensions and difficulties will arise where there are conflicting interests and it will take courage and practical moral wisdom to resolve these, if it is possible to do so (White 1985).

The moral problems in the remainder of this book will be examined in more detail in the light of the principles of beneficence, justice and respect for persons, and will be examined within a structure where we move from consideration of moral issues in direct nurse–patient relationships, to consideration of problems in nursing groups of patients and finally the wider responsibilities of nurses and society.

REFERENCES

Baric L 1974 Acquisition of the smoking habit and the model of smokers' careers. Journal of the Institute of Health Education 12, (1)

Boyd K M 1979 The ethics of resource allocation. Edinburgh University Press, Edinburgh

Campbell A V 1972 Moral dilemmas in medicine. Churchill Livingstone, Edinburgh

Campbell A V 1985 Paid to care. SPCK, London

Clough A H 1974 The latest decalogue. From: Poems Mulhauser F L (ed) Oxford University Press

Dorn N, Nortoft B 1982 Health careers, Institute for the Study of Drug Dependence, London

Ewles L, Simnett I 1985 Promoting health: A practical guide to health education. Wiley, Chichester

Goffman E 1961 Asylums. Anchor Books, New York

HMSO 1978 Report of Royal Commission on the National Health Service. HMSO, London

Illich I 1977 The limits of medicine. Penguin Books, Harmondsworth

McKeown T 1979 The role of medicine: Dream, mirage or nemesis. Blackwell, Oxford

Rumbold G 1986 Ethics in nursing practice. Baillière Tindall, London

Seedhouse D 1986 Health — the foundations for achievement. Wiley, Chichester

Thompson I E 1976 Suicide and philosophy. Contact 54

Thompson I E 1979 The nature of confidentiality. Journal of Medical Ethics 5 (2), 57–64

Thompson I E 1984a Ethical issues in palliative care. In: Doyle D Palliative care: The management of far advanced illness, Croom Helm, London, Ch 22

Thompson I E 1984b Ethical issues in community-based psychiatry. In Reed J, Lomas G Psychiatric Services in the Community: Developments and Innovations. Croom Helm, London, Ch 4

White R 1985 Political issues in nursing, Wiley, Chichester Vols 1 & 2

Wilson M 1976 Health is for people. Darton Longman & Todd, London

WHO 1947 Constitution of World Health Organization, United Nations Organizations, New York

WHO 1978 Primary Health Care: Report of the International Conference on Primary Health Care, Alma Ata, USSR. WHO, Geneva

WHO 1981 Regional Programme in Health Education and Lifestyles. Regional Committee for Europe, 31st Session, Berlin, EUR/RC31/10, WHO, Copenhagen

6

Moral dilemmas in direct nurse–patient relationships

6.1 Case-based discussion of ethics in nursing

In previous chapters we examined what we mean by moral problems and moral dilemmas, discussed how values come into the socialisation process of becoming and being a nurse, and explored how moral responsibility and accountability operate in the professional and institutional settings in which nurses work. In Chapter 4 we explored the implications of various models of power relationships and power sharing in nurse–patient relationships for an understanding of nursing ethics, and also discussed the fundamental principles of beneficence, justice and respect for persons as a basis for ethics. In Chapter 5 we looked at some of the classic big dilemmas in medicine, in the light of the following: our use of 'health' and 'disease' as value terms; the general trend towards the 'medicalisation' of life; and the concept of individual 'health careers'.

In this and the following two chapters we shall look at some of the specific moral problems and dilemmas faced by nurses in three different kinds of situations:

— In direct nurse–patient relationships
— In nursing groups of patients
— In the relationships of nurses to wider society.

In discussing direct nurse–patient relationships there are a number of approaches which could be adopted. For example, a traditional approach would be through an exploration of the concept of 'duty' and the specific duties of nurses. Alternatively, we could explore the scope and limits of an ethic of 'caring'. In this chapter we have chosen to approach the subject through an analysis of the rights of patients and how these relate to the duties of nurses, including the rights of nurses and the duties of patients. Although the approach we have adopted may have its limitations, we hope that we will be able to do justice to the concepts of 'duty' and 'caring' as well. However, it should be remembered that other approaches are possible.

We will discuss particular cases to illustrate some of the issues relating to the rights and duties of patients and nurses. In doing so, it will also become apparent that there are particular areas in which the rights and duties of nurses may come into conflict with those of medical staff, relatives or other nursing staff.

In discussing the issues which arise when nursing groups of patients, we will explore the moral responsibilities and moral dilemmas of management, teaching and research in nursing: conflicts between the rights of individual patients and the common good of other patients; the duty of nurses to provide a competent and efficient service for all in their care; and, the duty to maintain standards by research, education and training and professional integrity. The wider responsibilities of nurses in society are examined in Chapter 8, in particular issues of professional and public accountability; conflicts between the 'professional' and 'political' duties of the nurse, including the 'right' to strike; and the nurse as an agent of health and social policy.

This and the following two chapters will look at what is involved in making moral decisions in these types of situations, and attempt to clarify the issues. Moral decision-making is a problem-solving activity and skill, as will be discussed more fully in Chapter 9.

In applied ethics, and nursing ethics is a case in point, we look at typical cases of moral problems and dilemmas in the hope that we may learn from the way others have thought about or dealt with similar problems. In ordinary life, it is important that we should be able to learn from our own past experience. Similarly in nursing, the accumulated 'practical wisdom' or 'common sense' of the profession, our colleagues and wider society can give us some general guidance on how to act. However, this does not precisely tell us what to do in a particular situation. 'Casuistry' — or the study of cases and precedents — can be helpful, but does not decide things for us, any more than does the ward sister's anecdote of how she dealt with a 'similar' case. We have to decide for ourselves, but knowing what others have thought or done prevents us from having to 'start from scratch'

6.2 Institutional, legal and moral rights

It has become popular in the last 20 years to speak of 'patients' rights', and the American Hospital Association has codified a Bill of Rights for Patients (AHA 1973). However, it is also becoming common, in this context, to speak of the 'rights of nurses' as well. Rumbold (1986) devotes a whole chapter of his book to the discussion of the rights of nurses. But what do we mean by 'rights'? The term was introduced in Chapter 3.4 with a brief explanation, but at this point it is necessary to discuss it in more detail.

Broadly speaking, we may distinguish between institutional and legal rights on the one hand, and moral rights on the other. Consider the following example:

In Cleveland Health Authority, between January and July 1987, 110 children were taken into care by the social services, on the advice of two paediatricians, because of suspicions that these children were subject to sexual abuse at home. Legal representatives of the parents contested the *right* of the social services to take these children into care. In seeking leave to appeal to the High Court it was claimed that the *rights* of the parents had been infringed. Furthermore, it was claimed in evidence that the children had been subjected to several painful and humiliating examinations of their genitalia and other private parts, that repeated examinations involved violation of their *rights* (to privacy and respect for their persons), and that the doctors had not showed due care for these vulnerable patients. The local police surgeon complained that his *right* to be consulted by the paediatricians, before care orders were signed, had not been respected. Also at issue were the *rights* of the paediatricians, their right to examine the children and recommend they be taken into care, and their *right* to a fair hearing in the public enquiry.

In this case several parties claimed that their rights, or those of others, had been violated or infringed. However, if we look carefully at each use of the term 'right' or 'rights', we will see that they do not all mean the same thing. In the first instance the term clearly has a *legal* meaning, referring to the legal authority of the social services to issue care orders and to have children taken into care. This also applies to the authority of the paediatricians to examine the children. Here it is the legitimacy of their *authority* which is being questioned.

With reference to the parents' 'rights', the term is being used in a double sense — *both a legal and a moral sense.* The legal sense relates to whether their proper entitlement to a second medical opinion, or appeal to the High Court, has been taken into account. However, public interest in this case and the enquiry which followed, was stimulated by the insinuation in the press that the general moral rights of parents were at risk: such as their right of access to their own children. The rights of the children which it was claimed were not respected were fundamental *moral rights*, based on the principle of respect for persons — in particular their rights to privacy, dignity and proper care and treatment. What is of particular interest here is that the doctors and social workers claimed that they were exercising a proper duty-to-care in having the children medically examined and placed under care orders, to protect their rights, that is, to protect them from further sexual exploitation or abuse. What we have here is two different parties taking up the defence of the children and basing their arguments on appeal to different rights.

Finally, the right appealed to by the police surgeon is what may be called an *institutional right*, that is, an accepted protocol or courtesy exercised in the relationships of doctors, social workers and police. The rights of the paediatricians to a fair hearing would ordinarily be protected by institutional provisions for their legal representation by their employing authority, failing which they would be defended by the Medical Defence Union. However, their 'right' to a fair hearing could be said to be a right to which we are all entitled as a matter of natural justice, a fundamental moral right, but it is a right which may also be guaranteed in law, as a legal right as well.

Each of these different kinds of 'rights' has a different kind of justification. As we said in Chapter 5, in discussing voluntary euthanasia and the claimed right to die, 'Generally speaking moral and legal rights are justified claims that entitle us to demand that other people act or desist from acting in certain ways.' Rights which require people to desist from doing certain things to us, we call negative rights; and rights which entitle us to ask, or in some cases demand, that people do certain things for us, we call positive rights. In this sense rights impose on others *duties to do* things for us, or *duties not to do* things to us. These duties may be legally enforceable or may depend simply on the agent recognising the moral duty to act or desist from acting in a particular way. Because of this important practical connection between rights and duties, and the fact that we often have reciprocal rights and duties to others, it is important to understand that different kinds of rights will be subject to different kinds of justification.

Institutional rights are created by and can be abolished by decisions of people with competent authority. For example, the rule that only members of the Marylebone Cricket Club have the right to use the club facilities or to introduce visitors to the members' bar, will be decided by the elected and life members of the governing body of the MCC.

Legal rights must either be enacted by competent legal authorities, such as Parliament, regional or local authorities; or must be based on bills of rights such as the United Nations Universal Declaration of Human Rights or the American Constitution. Alternatively, they must be based on common or natural law, that is, the body of principle and precedent embodied in the legal tradition of the country. The first kind of legal rights, statutory rights, are explicitly stated in law, and in most cases are legally *enforceable* — in the sense that individuals can claim their rights or seek redress for the violation of their rights through the courts. The second kind, based on bills of rights, may be enforceable through appeal to an international agency such as the International Court of Human Rights, provided the country of the person making the appeal respects the authority of the higher court. However, these rights may be expressed in general terms and it would be the task of constitutional or international lawyers to interpret the constitution, or bill of rights, to see if the particular claim of the individual was justified in terms of the principles embodied in these statements of general rights. Claims based on common law, or principles of natural law, may also have to be interpreted in this way as both embody general statements of a moral rather than a legal kind. Their application in specific cases may have to be a matter of appeal to precedent, or some specific legislation may have to be introduced to make the principles applicable to the type of case in question.

In fact, if we consider the way that the term 'rights' is used in political life, in the general rhetoric of politicians and in the activity of pressure groups, it is significant that both are seeking as a rule to clarify or extend the scope of the law, or mobilise public opinion to change the law. Thus debate about the 'woman's right to choose' (to terminate a pregnancy on demand), or the 'right to employment', or the 'right to a living wage', or the 'right to free health care', or the 'rights of the unborn child', or 'the right to die' — are all concerned with the actual or possible reform of the law in the light of what people believe are their moral rights.

On what basis, then, do we justify moral rights? Generally, people appeal to their 'rights' when outraged by some injustice, or are protecting their human dignity when faced by degrading social conditions. In fact, appeal to moral rights presupposes the existence of fundamental moral principles, or at least a common intuition or consensus about fundamental moral principles. Thus appeal to 'the right to adequate care and treatment' or 'the right to protection' (for children, the old, the mentally and physically handicapped) is based on the assumption that society and the law will recognise the fundamental principle of beneficence (or the duty to care). The appeal to 'the right to equality before the law', to 'the right to freedom from discrimination on the basis of sex, class, religion or political affiliation', and the claimed 'right to equality of opportunity', or 'equal rights of access to health care', is based in each case on appeal to the fundamental principle of justice. Similarly appeal to individual rights, such as the 'right to know', the 'right to privacy' and the 'right to refuse treatment', is based in these cases on appeal to the fundamental principle of respect for persons.

In the broadest sense, the argument about human rights,

particularly universal moral rights, rests on appeal to some general concept of human dignity, that is, to some concept of what it means to be human, and what minimum conditions would have to be satisfied. In that sense, as we indicated in Chapter 4, sections 4 and 5, the definition of 'human nature' and 'natural law' can be expanded in certain universal moral principles and specific rights can be derived from these. Alternatively, if we argue that universal moral principles are decided by society on the basis of a kind of social contract or consensus, moral rights would be derivable, as practical implications, of these social contracts for the lives of ordinary people as moral agents. Whether human rights are 'inalienable', and in what sense, will depend on whether you believe that fundamental moral principles are God-given, grounded in the nature of things or determined by social convention. Whether human rights are to be regarded as 'absolute' will depend on similar considerations. However, there are two kinds of formal arguments which suggest that it is unhelpful to describe human rights as absolute. The first argument is that we should refer to the fundamental moral principles from which rights are derived as absolute, rather than the moral rights themselves. The second point is that in almost all cases of universal human rights, the exercise of their rights by one person may place limitations on the rights of others. Thus in the interests of justice our rights may have to be subject to limitation to protect the common good, for example the freedom of movement or association of people may have to be limited in times of war or epidemic.

It should be noted that in addition to general institutional, legal and moral rights there are specific rights of individuals arising out of private contracts or promises made: for example, marriage contracts, business contracts, bets, or promises to give money, services, to keep a secret. While these rights are not universal, as general legal and moral rights are, the moral principles underlying the keeping of contracts, promises, secrets are generally taken to be universally binding.

6.3 Rights and duties in nurse–patient relationships

If we consider practical examples of recurrent moral

dilemmas in nurse–patient relationships we shall see that many of these raise fundamental questions about the rights of patients and the scope and limits of the responsibilities of nurses. Such dilemmas as 'To tell or not to tell?', 'To treat or not to treat?', 'To limit the patient's freedom in his best interests?', and 'Which patient's interests or needs takes precedence?' all raise questions of this kind.

What, then, are the rights of patients, and how are they derived from the fundamental moral principles we have been discussing?

If we accept that there are such things as fundamental human rights, then it is important to note at the outset that patients' rights form a subclass of general human rights. If we would seek to ground human rights on principles of natural justice then patients' rights would be derived from general principles of natural law. We could start with the UN Universal Declaration of Human Rights and seek to expand these to cover the particular circumstances of health care. A third approach might be to start with the implicit assumptions of the contract-to-care between the carer and client, nurse and patient, and see what moral and legal implications there are of such contracts.

Here we shall adopt the approach of looking first at the way contractual obligations arise in consulting relationships, and then consider the moral assumptions on which these rest.

In general, when a person with a health problem seeks help they go first to a doctor. The doctor then decides on the form of care and treatment required, and either prescribes treatment directly, refers the 'patient' to hospital or specialist unit, or may refer the patient to a nurse for continuing care. Although it is increasingly common for patients to consult directly with nurses, particularly in community settings, nevertheless the 'contract-to-care' is usually made with the doctor, and the nurse has derived rather than direct duties following from the 'contract' with the 'patient'.

Despite these considerations, it may be useful to think through the process by which a person negotiates with a carer for help, and what the underlying assumptions are of agreements made. In general, the specific rights of people as 'patients' flow from the kind of relationship into which they enter with health-care staff. When a patient is lucid, ambulant, continent, and able to approach the health services independently for help, there is a kind of contract set up in which the patient agrees to co-operate in 'investigations', 'treatment' and 'rehabilitation', in return for appropriate 'therapy' and supportive care. The situation is rather different if the 'patient' is brought in unconscious, or is unconsultable because of the specific nature of his disease or injury, or by reason of mental disorder. Here the health professionals have to assume total responsibility for the 'patient' and must fall back on their own and their professional moral code for guidance. A third situation is where the carer is involved with the 'patient' as a friend — either through previous association, special circumstances of shared confidences, or because the person is dying and needs care and support rather than further therapy. Here the relationship may take on a more intimate form and the moral commitment in the contractual relationship may need to be renegotiated as something more personal and informal.

In Chapter 4 we described three different possible models for carer/client relationships, namely, Code, Contract and Covenant. Here we can see their application to the kinds of situations described. The ordinary situation where a person independently approaches the health services for help with a health problem is one in which an implicit or explicit contract-to-care is established by negotiation. In such a contract there will be rights and duties on the part of the patient and corresponding duties and rights on the part of the carer. In the second case, where the person is incompetent, the professional carer exercises a quasiparental and protective duty-to-care towards the vulnerable 'patient', governed by the code of practice of the profession. In the third type of situation, which we have suggested is governed by a covenant of friendship, special consideration may be given to the rights of the patient as a person, and the patient may feel able to make unusual demands on the carer in the knowledge that they are prepared to act 'over and beyond the call of duty'.

When a person approaches a doctor or other health professional for help, the carer has the right to refuse to help that particular person. They might legitimately refuse for several kinds of reasons. For example:

— If they have such a heavy caseload already that they could not provide adequate care and support
— If they do not believe they have the necessary competence
— If the person is being abusive and unpleasant, and they do not wish to have them as a client.

If a carer refuses a client on such grounds, they would be exercising their ordinary moral rights, but they would also have a professional duty to at least refer the person to someone else who might be able to help them with their problem.

Refusal in the first case would be justified on the grounds that the carer has the right not to be exploited or to have heavier demands imposed on them than they could reasonably be expected to cope with. Furthermore, carers have a duty, in justice to their clients, not to take on more clients than they could possibly provide with adequate care. So too, in the case of the difficult client, refusal to take them on may be in the client's best interests as well as the carer's. In these examples the rights in question would appear to be derivable mainly from considerations of justice, although respect for persons comes into it as well.

Once the carer agrees to take on the person seeking help, they acquire *fiduciary responsibility* for the client, that is, a responsibility to look after the client's interests and to protect their rights. This responsibility of the carer follows from the trust the client shows in the carer. In the standard consultation, the client is expected to give the carer appropriate information about themselves and their problems, to enable the carer to decide about the form of treatment to recommend. In a medical consultation, a doctor would not only take down a medical history but would probably proceed to physical examination, if this was required. Psychiatric assessment and a full social history may also be required. A nurse, in assessment of a patient and in order to develop a proper care plan, would quite likely follow a similar series of steps. The general assumptions underlying the exercise of these rights by the carer are that they are entitled to these privileges of intimacy because they are exercising a beneficent 'duty-to-care', in the best interests of the patient.

Although rather belatedly recognised, patients also have rights within these contracts-to-care. The Bill of Rights for Patients put forward by the American Hospital Association (AHA 1973) lists 12 rights of patients. The list is quite helpful in that it indicates areas where patients experience problems in dealing with health professionals. Attempts have been made to derive a simpler list from consideration of general contractual and moral rights. For example, Thompson (1975) suggested three fundamental rights of people as patients:

— The Right to Know
— The Right to Privacy
— The Right to Treatment.

People do not readily give others information of an intimate or private nature about themselves unless they expect some benefit from doing so. Patients, it has been argued, do not disinterestedly give doctors or nurses access to private information about themselves, nor allow intimate physical, psychological or social investigations without the expectation that the carer will give them in turn adequate information about how they propose to deal with the problem. The normal expectation of clients is that the carer will discuss their problem with them and give an opinion as to its nature; that the carer will discuss the proposed course of treatment or management of the problem; and that they will discuss the possible options and outcomes. Thus it can be argued that the right to know is implicit in the contract with the carer who is being consulted by the patient. Similarly, the requirement in law and medical ethics of informed and voluntary consent to treatment (unless the patient is incompetent) presupposes the patient's right to know. However, in this case the right to know tends to be based on wider considerations of the rights of the individual as a person (in the legal sense), that is, as someone who can be held responsible for their actions since they are capable of making informed and voluntary choices for themselves.

However, when a patient is dying or when news of a bad prognosis has to be communicated to a patient, health professionals may feel that they have a duty to protect the patient from knowledge which may be too painful to bear or which they are not yet ready to receive. In such cases there is a tension between the patient's right to know and the professionals' duty-to-care. How this tension is resolved in practice may vary from case to case. It may be further complicated by the intrusion of relatives who demand that the patient should not be told. In such cases, whose rights are to be given priority?

The right to privacy covers both the right to respect for the dignity of the person (physical privacy) and respect for secrets (confidentiality). The right to privacy does not mean the right to have a private ward, or the right to private medicine, although in some circumstances it may include that. For example, the elderly lady who has never shared a room with another person may be emotionally distressed at having to be nursed in a public ward, and might prefer to pay extra health insurance to ensure that she can get the privacy so important to her. The general loss of privacy may be expected by most people entering hospital, but it is also true that much of hospital care shows scant consideration for people's sensitivities or needs for privacy, particularly the dying.

Generally people are prepared to expose their secrets, expose their bodies and reveal their vulnerabilities when they need help and when they feel they can trust the person from whom they are seeking help. In such a situation, a sensitive carer will respect the patient's confidences and privacy. The carer will also recognise that the information is to be used only for the benefit of the patient, and that they thus acquire duties of advocacy, to protect the rights and interests of the person in their care, in the light of what they know about them.

The right to privacy, to have confidences kept, is not an unlimited right (UKCC 1984, clause 9). When the interests of justice require that evidence is brought before a court to establish the guilt or innocence of an accused it is generally assumed that the principle of justice and the common good takes precedence over the individual's right to privacy. In Britain, only lawyers enjoy 'professional privilege', that is, the right to refuse to disclose information in court (for example, information which may compromise the defence of a client). Priests and journalists, doctors and nurses do not enjoy this privilege, and if they refuse to divulge secrets of patients or penitents, which they may feel obliged to do, they may have to suffer the penalties for being 'in contempt of court'. In practice the court may not insist if the confidant is adamant, but as the law stands it is entitled to impose fines or send a person to prison for refusing to give evidence.

Similarly, when the public interest is threatened, for example by a serious epidemic, the nurse may be expected to divulge information to the responsible authorities if a patient's condition is likely to put the lives of other people at risk. In the context of the AIDS epidemic, if a nurse learns that a patient is having a sexual relationship with a person who is HIV-positive but is not prepared to disclose this to her doctor, what is the nurse to do? The patient's right to privacy may have to be compromised to protect others. Many other cases could be considered to illustrate the same moral dilemma in less dramatic circumstances, for example, the epileptic who discloses to the nurse that he is a long-distance lorry driver, or the 'unemployed' and 'disabled' patient who reveals to the district nurse that he is falsely claiming benefits when actually earning good money.

The disclosure of information to another health professional involved in his care may be expressly forbidden by a patient. But in certain circumstances, where the patient's safety or welfare is at stake, the nurse may decide, on the principle of beneficence, that her duty to care takes precedence over the patient's right to prohibit disclosure of vital facts (UKCC 1987).

A different kind of problem for the nurse arises because some people establish a kind of intimacy by sharing secrets and thus create a kind of obligation on the part of the nurse towards them, which they manipulate. Being at the receiving end of people's secrets can create burdensome problems for carers when, for example, the intimacies are irrelevant to the management of the problem. Similarly, health visitors, for example, can be faced with conflicts of duties when they discover on a domiciliary visit that the patient/client is concealing the true nature of his problem, or that he, or someone living with him, is breaking the law. Setting limits to confidentiality may be in the interests of both the patient and the nurse. The guidance given by the British Association of Social Workers to their members, namely that social workers should seek to establish explicit 'confidentiality contracts' with clients, remains fundamentally good advice for all professionals in consulting professions (BASW 1971).

While patients may share secrets in an attempt to gain some influence over their carers, it is also true that knowledge of their secrets gives professionals great power over people. This power can be used for the patient's benefit, but it can also be abused, for example as a means to get a patient to co-operate in treatment. The case of direct blackmail or breach of confidentiality are both serious offences and can lead to heavy penalties against professionals. However, the use of confidences as leverage to get patient compliance is more difficult to prove, and in some cases the carer may feel that the action is justified. Doctors and nurses are given great power to help or hurt people by the secrets they share with them, and with this power goes a great responsibility on the part of all those in the consulting professions (Thompson 1979).

Every person who has been taken on by a doctor or nurse as a patient has a right to expect proper care and treatment. The doctor or nurse is employed to provide a service, or offers a service on a fee-for-service basis, and the 'patient' is entitled to 'treatment' in fulfilment of the contract-to-care established when the doctor or nurse accepts them as a 'patient'. It might be argued on more general grounds that people have a fundamental human right to adequate health care (as in the UN Declaration of Human Rights, article 25), on the grounds that they cannot lead a full life without it. In Britain, the National Health Service Act of 1947 also created the legal right for citizens to claim medical treatment, which should be free at the point of delivery (although financed by general taxation). In reality the right to treatment is, for all practical purposes, based on the contract, formal or informal, between the particular doctor or nurse and a specific patient. This right is not absolute, however. The patient cannot demand whatever treatment they fancy even if they are in a position to pay for it. It is for the doctor or nurse to decide whether the treatment requested is appropriate. It also may not be possible to give a particular patient the special treatments which they request without detriment to the interests of other patients. Furthermore, while the patient has a fundamental moral right to adequate care and treatment, that 'treatment' may not be either drug therapy or surgery, or any other active intervention. In the case of the dying patient, 'treatment' may simply mean 'tender loving care' rather than therapy. The fact that the term 'treatment' covers both 'palliative care' and 'therapy' can be a source of confusion in discussions about 'stopping treatment'. While it may be appropriate to stop 'therapy', it would never be right to stop 'palliative care', such as the alleviation of pain or distressing symptoms.

In summary, there are three points which should be emphasised about patients' rights, as with human rights in general, namely:

— Having rights does not mean that one is bound to exercise them
— Having rights does not mean that their exercise is unlimited
— Negative rights are in general stronger than positive ones.

Thus having the right to know does not mean that one has to exercise it. One may not wish to know that one is dying, for example; or even if one suspects that one is dying, one may not wish to discuss it; or one may not wish to discuss it with a particular doctor or nurse. One has a right to be asked, but not obliged to accept unwanted information or 'counselling'. The right to privacy is not an unlimited right, because the demands of caring for others in similar need with limited staff and resources may require that patients sacrifice some of their privacy and consent to be nursed in public wards. While doctors and nurses are encouraged to regard respect for confidentiality as an important moral duty, it is generally recognised by hospital staff (and often by patients themselves) that team management necessitates the operation of a kind of 'extended confidentiality', which includes other members of the caring team. While the right to treatment is a fundamental right of patients, it does not include the right to demand particular therapies. However, the negative right to refuse treatment is a much stronger right. In law it is virtually an absolute right, unless the patient is mentally disordered, and the treatment of a patient against their will is technically a criminal assault and is actionable in law.

6.4 Telling the truth to patients or relatives

Consider the following situation faced by a young staff nurse in a paediatric hospital:

Mary, aged 13 years, was admitted with acute myeloid leukaemia. Over the next two and a half years she was in and out of hospital at increasingly frequent intervals. The permanent ward staff established a good relationship with Mary and her family during this period. Initially her parents did not accept the diagnosis, but with much support and reassurance eventually accepted the situation fairly well.

Two and a half years after her first admission, Mary was admitted for terminal care. Throughout the course of her illness her parents had been adamant that Mary should not be told what was wrong with her. This was still the situation when Mary was admitted for the last time. We tried to point out to her parents that Mary was no longer a child and that if the question of her condition arose, it might help her to know the truth, but they still refused to let her be told.

Three days before she died, Mary asked outright if she was going to die. She said she felt she was getting worse rather than better, and she asked directly what it was like to die.

In spite of her parents' views I felt that I had to be truthful with Mary as she was no longer a child, but 15 years old. We talked about death and I explained to her that everyone had to die sooner or later. I was with her when she died, as were her parents, and she died peacefully and calmly. I felt I had done the right thing in telling her, but felt that I had betrayed her parents' trust, which had been built up over nearly three years.

The staff nurse in this case recognised that knowing the truth that Mary was dying imposed certain responsibilities on her, to protect Mary's vulnerability (a feeling shared with Mary's parents), but she also recognised that Mary had a right to know the truth. The dilemma she faced was the conflict of loyalties to Mary and to her parents, because of the trust and understanding that had grown up between her and Mary on the one hand, and between her and Mary's parents on the other. The problem was made more difficult by her uncertainty that it was right to tell Mary, and her sense of guilt at going against the declared wishes of Mary's parents. She may also have been aware of having been specially chosen by Mary as the one to ask this momentous question. Was it not possible that the distraught parents, faced with loss of their daughter, were using the staff nurse in a vain attempt to re-assert their rights over their daughter? In such a situation, which does the nurse put first: the rights of the parents or the rights of the patient?

It is questionable whether doctors or nurses, or relatives ever have a right to keep information from a dying patient. Whose death is it anyway? If the dying patient does not have a fundamental right to know that they are dying, who has? However, in this case the patient was a child, 12 years old when myeloid leukaemia was first diagnosed, and only 15 when she died. Both the nurse and the parents assumed that they had a duty to protect Mary from the knowledge of her impending death, because she was a child. But did they have the right to deny her this knowledge? Because Mary was so young, at first the staff nurse felt initially that the parents were right to protect her from the painful truth, but as Mary grew older and asked more searching questions the staff nurse's attitude changed. However, did Mary have any more right to know at age 15 than at age 12? Are parents or relatives of dying patients entitled to withhold the truth from them however young or old they are?

In general, the right to know is derived from the principle of respect for persons. If people are to be treated as persons with · rights — for example, the right to make informed choices, the right to autonomy, that is, to be in control of their own lives — then they cannot be denied the knowledge or information which will enable them to make important life choices. We say glibly that 'Ignorance is bliss', but many studies show that dying patients are often frightened because they do not know what is going on, are aware of the conspiracy of silence around them, and are too afraid to ask. There is also evidence that dying patients are often reassured by knowing, as the anxiety based on doubt and uncertainty is ended, and in some cases their condition may improve spontaneously once they 'know the score' (Parkes 1966, Hinton 1979).

The policy of openness adopted by hospices for the dying is based not only on the belief that the patient has a right to know (particularly if he asks), but that good terminal care presupposes the knowing co-operation of the patient. The conspiracy of silence around the dying patient deceives no one — except perhaps the conspirators themselves. Several studies involving terminally ill patients have shown that in units where it is the policy not to tell, more than 75% of patients nevertheless do know that they are dying. Not surprisingly, patients pick up this information from various sources: by comparing their symptoms and treatment with other patients, by what they learn indirectly from conversation with other patients and hospital staff (including dinner ladies and porters), by observation of their own deteriorating condition and by what they infer from the body-language (non-verbal communication) of nurses and medical staff (hushed voices, telling looks, silent passing of the bed, over-solicitous care). The available evidence suggests that when told that their condition is terminal, patients do not 'give up', 'turn their faces to the wall', 'go to pieces', provided they are given adequate emotional support and time to come to terms with death.

However, it is not such pragmatic considerations which are of fundamental importance in this argument, but rather the fact that knowledge is power. Deliberately keeping another person in a state of ignorance is to deprive them of power, which results in a state of dependency and powerlessness. The attitude of Mary's parents had the effect of 'infantilising' her, depriving her of the opportunity to discuss with them her grief and anxiety at facing death. Their protective paternalism mirrors the attitudes often adopted by doctors and nurses in being more concerned to protect the patient than to respect their rights as persons to know and choose for themselves.

Consider another case:

A nurse midwife is caring for a mother who has had a stillborn baby, by caesarian section, just recovering consciousness and asking to see her baby. How, when and where does the nurse tell the mother that her baby is dead? Should she call for the doctor and get around the difficulty that way? Should she tell the absent father first? Should she avoid telling the mother till the father is present and can comfort his wife? Should she arrange for the couple to see the baby? How does she cope with her own grief, her own feelings of failure, her need to appear strong in order to comfort the parents and to continue providing care to the mother?

In this case, the mother not only has a right to know, but is bound to know sooner or later. The grief cannot be avoided. The question is whether the nurse can cope with being the one who tells, who shares the mother's grief and the mother's likely sense of her own failure, and who is available to provide on-going support afterwards. The inhibition which the nurse feels about sharing the truth in this situation, particularly if there is no convenient way out of facing the challenge, probably has more to do with her fear of accepting the responsibility for telling the truth, than any uncertainty about the mother's rights. Sharing the truth can be a costly business. Once the midwife accepts the *responsibility* to tell the mother she implicitly commits herself to share her grief (and with the husband perhaps). If she knows anything about loss and bereavement she will also know that telling parents that a longed-for baby has died will not only cause them immediate grief but will initiate a process which may take many months to work through. She will also know that she has a duty to continue with support for as long as possible, while they deal with their bereavement. Truth-sharing means accepting responsibility to share the pain and grief, anger and despair, shock and depression which knowing the truth may cause. If there is not well-established understanding, trust and caring, if there is no possibility that the nurse can provide continuing support to the individual concerned, then 'telling the truth' may be cruel and irresponsible (Thompson 1984).

Sharing painful truth requires great sensitivity and skill in judging how, when and where it is appropriate to tell. Once the midwife accepts the responsibility to tell the mother, she also has to face the difficult practical decisions, requiring tact and judgement, whether the mother will be most helped by being allowed to cuddle her dead baby, or needs to be protected from an experience which may be too painful for her to bear or for which she is not yet ready. Being *honest* with other people is a measure of how much we trust and respect them as persons, how much we *honour* them. Honesty, or truthfulness, is being sensitive to 'where other people are at', in their own present experience and ability to cope. In making an assessment of a patient the nurse will not only have to rely on her own judgement and common sense, but on the opinions of her colleagues and perhaps the relatives. But the nurse can never shelve her responsibility by relying on, or being tied by, the opinions of others. Sooner or later all nurses have to face situations where they have to accept responsibility for sharing the painful truth with patients, and this means becoming as skilled in 'titrating' the truth to the needs of the patient as administering appropriate doses of pain-killing drugs.

A different but related problem about sharing information arises when the patient knows the truth yet refuses to let the medical or nursing staff tell his wife or family. Here in no direct sense do the relatives have a *right* to know since it is not their death that is at issue; but as people who are intimately involved and likely to be affected by the patient's death, the nurse may feel that they ought to be told. As we do not exist in isolation from other people, least of all our families, they have a right to know in an extended sense, based both on considerations of compassion and the reciprocal responsibilities which obtain in families and close communities.

Faced with such a situation, the nurse may be helped by discussing the matter with the person prohibiting the disclosure of information, to make them aware of how the interests of others are involved, to help them see what comfort may be gained by sharing the truth and the grief together. For example, Mary's parents might have been persuaded to tell Mary themselves (with or without the support of the medical and nursing staff); the husband might be persuaded and assisted to tell his wife about the baby himself, with the midwife providing support; the dying patient might need to be encouraged and assisted to share his anxieties about dying with his wife and family and to set his affairs in order. However, if they still refuse, the nurse may be able to gain moral support from discussion with other members of staff. But in the end, the nurse may have to make her own painful decision whether to tell. Here she has to balance several conflicting interests and duties: her responsibility to her patient against her wider responsibilities to the family and other concerned parties.

In the cases considered, it can readily be seen that dilemmas about truth-telling relate to the rights of patients (for example, the right to know and the right to privacy) and to the tensions between these rights and the duties of nurses (for example, the duty to protect the vulnerable patient from knowledge too painful to bear or the duty, in fairness to others, to share information that may affect them). Here we see that considerations other than respect for persons and their individual rights come into play. The principles of beneficence and justice are also involved, and it is precisely this actual or apparent conflict of principles which makes these present as moral dilemmas, and which makes decisions in these areas difficult, painful and uncertain.

6.5 Deciding between therapeutic care and palliative care

As already indicated, the right to treatment is a fundamental right of people as patients, regardless of their age or whether they can speak for themselves. The least problematic situation is where an independent adult, in full possession of his senses, enters into a contract for treatment with a doctor, or the caring team, when he becomes their patient. In principle, infants, the mentally handicapped, and elderly patients have the same rights and are entitled to the same standards of medical and nursing care as anyone else. When, by reason of physical or mental illness, a patient is in a very dependent and vulnerable condition, decisions have to be taken about care and treatment by others. The lucid, independent and ambulant patient can actively claim his right to treatment — or refuse treatment. The confused or unconscious, bedbound or unconsultable patient is a different matter, depending entirely on others to protect his rights and dignity, to ensure that he gets adequate medical treatment and proper nursing care. The infant born with serious physical or mental defects also needs to have his interests safeguarded. Just as special tribunals are set up to oversee the care and management of compulsory psychiatric patients, so the courts have a special responsibility to protect the rights of others who are not competent to defend themselves, owing to physical or mental infirmity, old age or infancy.

These safeguards are not because health-care workers cannot be trusted to care for their patients in a responsible fashion, but because they need protection as much as their vulnerable patients do, from criticism and litigation or worse. The unconsultable patient needs an independent advocate to represent his interests where there may be doubt and uncertainty about the right course of treatment or conflict between doctors and nurses, for example, about whether the patient's rights have been protected.

Part of the difficulty centres around the ambiguity of the word 'treatment', when we speak of the 'right to treatment'. If 'treatment' embraces medical interventions and nursing care, therapeutic measures and palliative care, compulsory hospitalisation and asylum, then it is important to be clear about what treatment is being referred to in a particular context. In certain contexts the purpose of an operation may be to cure, by repairing injury, removing diseased tissue or preventing the spread of infection. In another context surgery may be purely palliative, to relieve pain or to delay the spread of malignant disease. Alternatively, the operation may be strictly unnecessary for medical reasons, but indicated for psychological or social reasons, as, for example, cosmetic surgery, sterilisation or sex change. In each case, the 'right to treatment' will mean slightly different things.

Because 'treatment' means both 'cure' and 'care', it may in practice be difficult to separate the one from the other. When a patient has a potentially fatal disease, which might be curable or at least treatable, it may be extremely difficult for the ward team to decide when further therapeutic measures are no longer justified and it is time to 'settle for comfort'. For the caring team to be clear about when a patient has reached the pre-death stage is vitally important for good terminal care. But if a change of management to palliative care is indicated, the patient, it may be argued, has a right to be consulted about this step. A 'conspiracy of silence' about the true situation may also lead to conflict between nursing staff and doctors about which type of 'treatment' is appropriate. This may be particularly difficult if the patient or relatives are desperately demanding that everything possible should be done, or that all treatment should be stopped.

Consider the following three situations described by nurses:

a. When I was a student midwife, a baby with Down's syndrome and a severe heart defect was born to a 38-year-old mother and a 42-year-old father. Both parents were unable to accept the baby. The father expressed the wish that the baby should not be resuscitated if a crisis occurred. This happened soon afterwards and a junior member of the medical team initiated resuscitation. The baby died, however, several weeks later.

b. In my second year of nursing, during my second spell of night duty as a staff nurse, Margaret was admitted to our ward. She was 23 years old and recently married. She was suffering from oesophageal varices, and the consultant surgeon had used a new technique of portal-caval shunt in an attempt to treat her condition. Margaret's condition deteriorated after the operation and she was in considerable pain. The surgeon insisted she be kept completely drug-free to rest her liver, and the resident doctor consequently refused to sign her up for any pain-killing drugs, and instructed me to give a placebo only (whether intravenous or intramuscular). Margaret was in considerable pain and had more and more distressing nights. She was a most charming person and the staff were very fond of her. This made it very difficult for us, feeling we could not help. In the mornings the ward sister would come on duty, often very early and would demand to know whether Margaret had been sedated. When I told her that I had not been allowed to give her any sedation she would become very angry with me and would (to my relief) instruct me to give her sedation. Each day the same battle would go on between the consultant, resident, ward sister and myself — with the nurses concerned to make Margaret as comfortable as possible, and the consultant concerned that his operation should be a success. The battle continued until very close to Margaret's death, when the consultant surgeon finally conceded that she should be given adequate sedation.

c. While nursing in Accident and Emergency, a child victim of a road traffic accident, with severe injuries and loss of blood, was brought in by ambulance. The child's parents were Jehovah's Witnesses, and insisted that the child should not be given blood transfusions. The parents were asked to wait while X-rays were taken and other tests made. While these were being done it became apparent that the child would not survive without immediate blood transfusions. The child was given the necessary transfusion but the parents were not informed. The child survived.

In (a), the case of the Down's syndrome baby with a congenital heart defect, there are broadly speaking two schools of thought — the one that emphasises the rights of the baby and the one that emphasises the responsibility of the medical team. In principle, the baby has the same right to life and right to treatment that any adult has, and the law should safeguard these rights as it does those of other vulnerable individuals. An outside party (e.g. a social worker) should have the right to appeal to the courts to ensure that the child's rights are protected. Although all citizens have a moral duty to protect the rights of others — thus protecting their own rights — certain professionals, such as social workers and hospital chaplains, have special responsibility to act as advocates for those whose rights may be compromised or neglected. The parents do not have a moral right to refuse the treatment that their child requires for survival, but nor can they be forced to care for the child. If we recognise that the child has a right to treatment, then we must also recognise that society has an obligation to provide adequate care and support for the child (and possibly for the parents as well).

In practice, the situation is more complicated. The social provision for the care of severely handicapped children is inadequate, and support for affected families insufficient to prevent hardship and distress. Compassion for the parents, who, understandably, may feel unable to cope, and compassion for the medical and nursing staff, who are faced with immediate decisions about care and treatment for the child, may point to 'letting nature take its course' and allowing the child to die. In reality, the hospital team and the parents have to try to resolve the situation in the most responsible way. The risks of medical intervention are that the child would still be left severely handicapped for life, and would require constant nursing care and medical attention. The parents would almost inevitably have to carry the main burden of caring for the child because of the lack of practical alternatives.

Issues of social justice are involved as well, because the painful reality is that the child's right to treatment and the medical team's duty to care have to be reconciled in most cases where there is inadequate social provision for the care and support of such children and their families. This places unjust pressure on the family to accept responsibilities greater than they can cope with on their own, and pressure on the medical team who may not feel free to do what is in the child's best interests. This illustrates how issues of rights cannot be separated from considerations of justice relating to the equitable distribution of resources in society generally.

Clinical decisions in such cases are not unambiguous. Past experience may show that there is little hope for such children, or that particular interventions can be successful in ensuring survival and a reasonable quality of life. However, medical evidence will not be enough to resolve the moral dilemmas. How objective are assessments of 'quality of life'? How does one judge that a life of severe physical or mental handicap is better or worse than no life at all? We might set up criteria and tests of competence and capacity for independent living, but they may palpably fail to take account of the patient's own view of things — even if this is possible. A survey of adults with mental handicap in Scotland, found, contrary to prevailing opinion among medical policy-makers and managers of large institutions for the mentally handicapped, that over 75% of those in long-stay care would be capable of living in the community with minimal support (Baker & Urquhart 1987). There are considerable risks in depending on one group of professionals to define what 'quality of life' means for other people. Where the political will to provide adequate 'community care' is lacking, there is the additional risk that medical opinion will be used to rationalise the detention of mentally hadicapped people in special asylums for life.

The infant with Down's syndrome certainly had a right to treatment, but it does not follow that everything possible has to be tried, including the most expensive, untried or dangerous treatments. Treatment may mean direct interventions which aim to cure, or it may mean simply the provision of good nursing care and control of symptoms. Deciding which is appropriate in such a case may be difficult and morally ambiguous. It may be tempting to simply 'treat' the parents' distress or the ward team's anxiety by removing the object that is the cause, but that would not represent the kind of moral initiative the situation demands — the courage to act in spite of the practical uncertainty and moral ambiguity and to live with the consequences.

The distinction drawn by moral theologians between 'ordinary' and 'extraordinary' means is often invoked to deal with such situations. The health care team are obliged to give the child in such a case the 'ordinary' means of assistance but are not obliged to employ 'extraordinary' means in an attempt to save its life. However, it is doubtful that this distinction solves the moral dilemma in such cases, but points to the need for decisions to be based on common sense and due regard for the circumstances and needs of the patient and all parties with a responsibility to care. 'Leaving nature to take its course' seldom means doing nothing more for the affected infant; it would normally mean continuing to give fluids (and possibly food or drugs to suppress hunger) and keeping the infant comfortable and painfree. But it could also mean not intervening actively to give antibiotics, not performing an operation with a poor record of success, and not resuscitating the infant should it suffer cardiac arrest.

In the case we are considering, the houseman acted decisively to resuscitate the child, but she died anyway. His action was a perfectly understandable one. It was one possible response to a distressing situation, one possible attempt to resolve the painful dilemma. It was an action which had its own possible medical and moral justification. The child did after all survive for several weeks, and this may have been of some help to the parents in coming to terms with their bereavement. However, it might have been no less morally courageous, and possibly more difficult in the face of the pressure to 'do something!', to have left the child to die. Such situations are called dilemmas precisely because there is no way one can know with certainty, or unambiguously, what is the right thing do in the circumstances (Stinson & Stinson 1981).

Not taking any action to resuscitate a patient who has suffered cardiac arrest or choked is sometimes referred to as *passive euthanasia*, in contrast to *active euthanasia* when someone takes direct action to end the life of a patient. Some philosophers argue that there is an important moral distinction between active killing and letting someone die, in terms of the different intentions of the agent, and that while active euthanasia is not morally acceptable, in some circumstances passive euthanasia may be. Others argue that if the doctor or nurse knows that the patient will die as a result of discontinuing life support, this amounts to the same thing. The consequences are identical, the patient dies: the intentions 'to kill' or 'to deprive of life support' are virtually indistinguishable. There are complex and important arguments on both sides, but medical and nursing staff, faced with decisions to stop treatment or not to intervene, tend to maintain that there is a valid commonsense distinction between actively killing a patient (with or without the patient's consent), and taking no action to save his life when he is dying.

This so-called commonsense distinction between active and passive euthanasia, as well as the distinction between ordi-

nary and extraordinary means, is put under strain when we consider what has been made possible by the development of modern drugs, new anaesthetics and life-support machines. To some extent, the boundaries between 'ordinary' and 'extraordinary' means are changing all the time with the development of more sophisticated techniques and knowledge (as, for example, the definition of 'viability' has had to be changed from 28 weeks for neonates as it has proved possible to keep younger babies alive). These changes in the boundaries do not make decisions in these cases any easier. The presence or absence of sophisticated resuscitative equipment can make all the difference as to how a case is viewed. Is actively switching off a life-support system to a brain-dead patient being kept 'alive' for transplant purposes, active or passive euthanasia? Or neither? With more precise medical and legal criteria for defining death this particular dilemma may be removed, but with live and conscious patients who are dying the problems remain (Harris 1981).

In case (b), the conflict between the nurses and the doctors over the level of pain-control to be given to Margaret, we encounter a common problem in doctor/nurse relationships in terminal care. The problem relates to the different functions of the nurse and the doctor, and their perceived roles in relation to the severely ill patient — the nurse being more concerned with the comfort and well-being of the patient, the doctor with sorting out the medical problems. However, conflicts also tend to arise in the pre-terminal stage when it is as yet unclear whether the patient is dying or her life could be saved. While there is hope, curative measures are appropriate, even to the point of denying pain-killers if these may jeopardise the possibility of a cure. Once the situation is recognised to be hopeless in therapeutic terms, then appropriate palliative care should be given. Deciding when it is appropriate to switch from therapeutic to palliative measures may be difficult and fraught with uncertainty for the doctor, faced with possible charges of negligence if he misses something. The anxiety of the medical staff not to be found wanting drives them to do all they can, while the anxiety of the nursing staff at having to cope with the distress of the patient (and relatives) may drive them to demand that they should 'settle for comfort'. The doctor's experience that patients (especially young patients) may sometimes be 'snatched from the jaws of death' has to be balanced by the insight of experienced nurses that patients have 'turned the corner never to return'. Decisions about the type of management appropriate may have to be taken under pressure from rebellious nurses, or by the doctor asserting his medical authority. But decisions do have to be taken by someone, and that usually is the doctor, because of his ultimate legal responsibility.

A common dilemma in such circumstances relates to the use of powerful pain-controlling drugs such as diamorphine, which nevertheless can have dangerous side-effects — such as suppressing respiration — which may hasten the patient's death or make them more susceptible to infections which may kill them. Some nurses object to giving diamorphine to dying patients even if they are in great pain, because they regard this as a form of euthanasia. Even more nurses are afraid of being the one who administers the last injection and appearing to be responsible for the death of the patient. Clearly, the nurse has a moral right to refuse to do something which violates her conscience, but she may not have a legal right to refuse to carry out doctor's orders.

The 'principle of double effect' has sometimes been invoked to help provide commonsense guidance for action in such circumstances. When a nurse is confronted with a situation demanding action which she can forsee will have two effects, one good (such as relieving a patient's pain) and the other bad (putting the patient at risk of earlier death), she would be justified in performing the action subject to the following conditions, to quote from O'Keeffe (1984):

1. The action must itself be a good action, or at least morally neutral
2. The performance of the action must bring about at least as much good as evil
3. The evil effect must not be a means to achieving the good effect
4. The agent must have a justifying and sufficient reason for acting rather that refraining from acting.

It may be doubted whether these conditions entirely solve the dilemma, but they may help some people to cope with the painful responsibility involved. Better knowledge of pain control, and experience gained in terminal care units, has shown that proper use of diamorphine and other drugs not only greatly improves the quality of life of the dying patient, but can actually give them the strength and determination to live longer.

Case (c), the case of the child of Jehovah's Witness parents, raises in an acute form the question of whether parents have the right to decide for their children in such vital matters as those affecting their right to life, whether the parents' authority can override the ordinary rights of the child as a human being. So far as the law is concerned, the child does have the same right to life as an adult, and in most societies the courts can overrule the authority of parents — as in proven child abuse, or where the child might die if denied essential medical treatment. In this case, the medical and nursing staff colluded in deceiving the parents so as to ensure that the child was given the necessary life-saving blood transfusions. They might have applied to a judge and had the child made a ward of Court, and this might have been a more proper procedure, not least to protect themselves from litigation. (Although proxy consent-to-treatment by parents is often accepted on behalf of a child, by hospital authorities, the law is not clear on whether proxy consent is legally adequate, let alone morally acceptable) (McCormick 1976, Ramsey 1976, 1977). However, even with proper legal authority, the action of the medical team in this case leaves room for serious difficulties. Given the beliefs held by Jehovah's Witnesses, there was a risk that if the parents found out about the blood transfusion they would subsequently reject the child. If they did, the question would arise as to who would be responsible for the ongoing care of the child.

Where such a clash of values between parents and professionals takes place, the interpretation of rights and responsibilities becomes a matter of disagreement. The medical and nursing staff in such a situation should ideally make their own moral and legal viewpoint clear to the parents, and attempt to persuade them to accept the necessity for treatment while trying to accommodate their wishes where possible by the use of other measures, if these are available. However, if no other course is open to them, the medical and nursing staff may have to act against the parents' wishes, and they have a right to expect that the courts and society would give them and the child the necessary support.

148 / *Nursing Ethics*

REFERENCES

American Hospital Association 1973 A bill of rights for patients. American Hospital Association, New York
Baker N, Urquhart J 1987 The balance of care for adults with a mental handicap in Scotland. ISD Publications, Edinburgh
BASW 1971 Confidentiality in social work. British Association of Social Workers, London
Harris J 1981 Ethical problems in the management of some severely handicapped children. Journal of Medical Ethics 7 (3), 114–117
Hinton J 1979 Comparison of places and policies for terminal care. Lancet i, 6 January 29
McCormick R 1976 Experiments in children: sharing sociality. Hastings Center Report No. 6, 41–46
O'Keeffe T M 1984 Suicide and self-starvation. Philosophy, July
Parkes C M 1966 The patient's right to know the truth. Proceedings of the Royal Society of Medicine 66, 536
Ramsey P 1976 The enforcement of morals: Non-therapeutic research on children. Hastings Center Report No. 6, 29–31
Ramsey P 1977 Children as research subjects: A reply. Hastings Centre Report No. 7, 40–42
Rumbold G 1986 Ethics in nursing practice. Baillière Tindall, London
Stinson R, Stinson P 1981 On the death of a baby. Journal of Medical Ethics 7 (1), 5–18
Thompson I E 1975 Dilemmas of dying: A study in the ethics of terminal care. Edinburgh University Press, Edinburgh, Ch 5
Thompson I E 1979 The nature of confidentiality. Journal of Medical Ethics 5, 57–64
Thompson I E 1984 Ethical issues in teminal care. In: Doyle D (ed) Palliative care: The management of far advanced illness. Croom Helm, London, Ch 22
UKCC 1984 The Code of Professional Conduct for the Nurse, Midwife and Health Visitor, 2nd edn. United Kingdom Central Council for Nursing, Midwifery and Health Visiting, London
UKCC 1987 Confidentiality. United Kingdom Central Council, London

7

Moral dilemmas in nursing groups of patients

7.1 Responsibility for individuals and for groups of patients

The previous chapter discussed two classes of moral dilemma in direct nurse–patient encounters; these centred on dilemmas of truth-telling and confidentiality on the one hand, and dilemmas of deciding between therapeutic and palliative treatment on the other. While these dilemmas could not be discussed entirely without regard to the rights of other patients and relatives, the second two groups of moral dilemmas cannot be discussed without taking account of the rights of other patients or the good of society. These are dilemmas which relate to: setting limits to the 'management' of patients, that is, the control and direction of their lives; balancing the rights of individual patients with those of other patients, or third parties. It may be useful in this connection to distinguish a little more clearly between four different, but related senses of responsibility:

> Responsibility *for* one's own actions (personal responsibility)
> Responsibility *for* the care of someone (fiduciary responsibility)
> Responsibility *to* higher authority (professional accountability)
> Responsibility *to* wider society (public accountability/civic duty)

Personal responsibility. Ordinarily one is held responsible for one's own actions and praised or blamed for them, provided one knows what one is doing, has acted freely and voluntarily and provided one can distinguish between right and wrong. This sense of responsibility applies to all one's actions and is the most basic sense involved when one is being tried for negligence by a court or investigating inquiry. Here, excusing conditions which may be taken into account in determining the degree of guilt involved are: ignorance, stress of circumstances, inexperience in making moral decisions of the kind in question. (See chapter 9.5 and 9.6.)

Fiduciary responsibility. When someone is entrusted to your care (e.g. a child, an unconscious or mentally disordered patient), or when a patient voluntarily entrusts his life into your hands, whether as a nurse or in the context of lay care, you acquire fiduciary responsibility. Thus having responsibility for the care and treatment of patients, or for decisions about their individual and collective well-being, is a matter of fiduciary responsibility, and the power or authority of the nurse to do these things derives from the trust which the patient and society places in her.

Professional accountability. Because of the responsibility vested in nurses by patients and society, and underwritten in Britain by the National Board for Nursing Midwifery and Health Visiting (NBS) and the United Kingdom Central Council for Nursing Midwifery and Health Visiting (UKCC), nurses have a professional obligation or duty to give account of their actions to their peers, their superiors, to the NBS and UKCC, and to society through the courts, if necessary. This duty of professional accountability follows from the responsibilities entrusted to the nurse, as a nurse. Many nurses will feel both responsible for and responsible to their patients, and to relatives as well. Because the nurse is responsible for the patient's well-being, she may feel guilty if things go wrong and consider that some kind of explanation or apology is due to the patient or relatives. The sentiment might be right, and in some circumstances explanations or apologies might be in order, but it can also be inappropriate for the individual nurse to apologise or offer explanations, as this might also expose the nurse to prosecution for negligence in cases where the patient has suffered hurt or injury. The line of accountability in nursing must, in the first instance, be upwards to the line manager, then to the profession, as these authorities would be in a better position to decide whether a personal apology is due, or whether the issue should be dealt with through the appropriate complaints procedures. In some cases it will not be helpful (or wise) for nurses to give all the reasons for their actions to patients and relatives — at least not until demanded to do so by an enquiry. However, from the daily Kardex meeting and meetings of the medical care team through to enquiries by the disciplinary committees of the NBS and UKCC and the courts, nurses are obliged to give account of themselves, by virtue of the trust vested in them.

Public accountability/civic duty. The nurse is a member of a public body with corporate responsibilities. As a professional member of the National Health Service staff, the nurse has responsibility for maintaining the general standards of nursing care. As members of a profession committed to the care of patients, nurses have responsibilities to influence health policy and the allocation of resources. Nurses are public officers, even public servants, with both civic and political duties. They have individual civic responsibility to society to draw attention to specific examples of incompetence or negligence, or where standards of care have become unacceptable. They have public or political responsibility to act corporately, through nursing unions or associations, to try to bring about changes in practice, improved standards of care, more appropriate allocation of resources, more relevant health policies for the benefit of patients in general.

When nurses are compelled to weigh their responsibility for individual patients against their responsibilities for groups of patients, conflicts may arise between these different responsibilities which the nurse carries as a professional. The authority vested in her, to serve the best interests of her patients, may contrast with the actual or relative lack of power which she has — depending on her relationships with other staff, her position in the nursing hierarchy, what she is entitled to do by law, and what she is or is not allowed to do by her union or professional associations. Some of these dilemmas of responsibility and authority are among those to which we now turn.

7.2 Setting limits to the control and direction of patients

The management of patients is a complex art, ranging from subtle persuasion to the use of force to subdue violent patients. What gives the nurse the authority to control other people in this way?

In psychiatric wards, in accident and emergency departments and in working with people with mental handicaps, nurses often encounter violent patients who have to be restrained by physical means, by the use of drugs or by invoking the law. In such cases it may appear that the nursing staff are justified in using force to control patients simply in order to defend themselves and to defend other patients and staff. They may also be acting to protect the patient from injury, self-mutilation or suicide, or, less dramatically, 'acting in the patient's own best interests' (COHSE 1977).

The fact is that the nurse is not only responsible for the individual patient and his needs, nor solely concerned with his rights. The nurse also has to protect the interests of other patients and, as a public officer who is accountable to society at large, has to consider the public good. The rights of individual patients may have to be restricted where the rights of other people are put at risk. In addition, the nurse has a responsibility to protect the interests of the patient who is incapable of understanding what his own best interests are, e.g. if he is mentally ill, intoxicated or mentally handicapped. The nurse has to decide what is in the best interests of the patient and good patient care. Depending on the status of the patient, and the circumstances in which the patient comes or is referred to the nurse for appropriate care, nurses may interpret their responsibilities differently. (See Chapter 4.2 for a discussion of models of responsibility based on code, contract and covenant.) In general, nurses exercise fiduciary responsibility for patients entrusted to their care, and they must be guided in their decisions by training and experience, professional code and personal conscience, 'Acting always in such a way as to promote and safeguard the well-being and interests of patients/clients' (UKCC 1984).

Concern with the 'common good' and the 'best interests of the patient' means that the nurse exercises both clinical and moral responsibilities towards her patients. These responsibilities are determined not only by consideration of the patients' rights and respect for their freedom, but also by consideration of the wider health needs of the individual and the community. 'Management' of patients (including those who co-operate fully in treatment) can involve various degrees of control, ranging from physical restraint or legal measures, to behavioural modification, health education and simply directive managerial communication. Skill in nursing means, in part at least, learning to control people in the nicest possible way.

Moral responsibility and personal freedom

Consider the following problem encountered by a psychiatric nurse:

On our ward we had a 70-year-old woman who was described as an alcoholic and had taken several overdoses over a period of two years. The staff feared that if she were to be discharged she would return home to her alcoholic husband and sooner or later would be found dead. However, when she was sober she appeared completely rational and demanded to be allowed home. Her compulsory detention in hospital on the grounds that she might commit suicide seemed to me a flagrant violation of her freedom when there did not appear to be adequate evidence that she was mentally ill.

The same nurse went on to ask whether a nurse has a duty to prevent someone from committing suicide if they want to do so.

As long as a person is in the nurse's care, the law requires the nurse to protect them from harm and that includes self-inflicted harm. In fact, a nurse can be charged with negligence if a patient succeeds in killing himself. The nurse has this legal duty towards patients in her care in spite of the fact that suicide is no longer illegal. The law assumes that the instinct for self-preservation is natural in man and that acts of self-destruction indicate that 'the balance of a person's mind has been disturbed'. As mentally unbalanced, they are not prosecuted but nevertheless health professionals are expected to care for them and protect them from themselves. Most religions and virtually all human societies disapprove of suicide and therefore most nurses also feel a moral obligation to prevent people from killing themselves (Thompson

1976). The fact that the law allows people the licence or liberty to attempt suicide without prosecution does not mean that the law or morality recognises that persons have a *right* to kill themselves. We ordinarily understand by a 'right' the entitlement to demand that other people either assist us in particular ways or desist from acting towards us in particular ways. In this sense of 'right', the so-called 'right-to-suicide' is not a right; there is no way we can appeal to the law or to morality to compel others to assist us to end our lives. Whether we can extend the use of the term 'right' to cover personal entitlement to act in a particular way, for example, to attempt suicide, will depend on our understanding of the reciprocal obligations we owe one another, as members of the moral community. In general, society disapproves of suicide, not only because of the apparent contradiction between suicide and the instinct on which the right to life is based, but also because of the grief and hurt which it causes to others in society.

In the above mentioned case the ambiguity arises because of uncertainty about the elderly woman's mental state. Was she capable of making rational decisions about her life? The action of the hospital in protecting her might appear paternalistic and restrictive of her liberty, but it could be said to be a natural extension of her right to treatment and the contract of the staff to care for her (as well as to offer her such therapy as might be appropriate). Here the nurse has to exercise fiduciary responsibility on behalf of the patient and that may involve restricting her movements, 'in her own best interests' — a demand of protective beneficence and advocacy or defence of the patient's rights where the patient appears unable to take responsible decisions for herself. Of course, this argument presupposes that suicide is never in the best interests of the patient. The moving play Whose Life Is It Anyway?, about a young quadraplegic who is being kept alive against his will, by artificial means, challenges this assumption — at least as far as the young man is exercising his right to refuse further treatment and be left to die (Clark 1978).

A less generous construction which could be placed on the action of the hospital is that the staff were acting less to protect the old lady than to protect themselves against the charge of negligence and the guilt which might result if the patient succeeded in killing herself. The fact is, that no matter what precautions are taken, some patients do succeed in committing suicide and that does cause great distress to the staff responsible for their care. Nevertheless, defensive action and conservative measures, though somewhat repressive at times, are not morally unjustifiable. On the contrary, staff are entitled to protect themselves and their professional reputations. The courage to take the risk of discharging a potentially suicidal patient may show admirable regard for their autonomy but can always be attacked as irresponsibility. Achieving a balance between caring for and protecting patients and respecting their freedom, between defensive medicine and attempted rehabilitation, is always difficult, a matter of risk and often complicated by the threat of legal action.

Behaviour modification

Another type of control which raises ethical problems is the use of rewards and punishments to reinforce behaviour modification in long-term psychiatric patients. For example, money or cigarettes may be given as rewards to encourage better self-care among institutionalised patients — for washing, shaving, dressing, bed-making, care of living area; and sanctions may be applied — by the removal of privileges such as access to television, opportunities for exercise or recreation. Is it ethically justifiable to extend the definition of treatment to include the retraining and rehabilitation of patients by these means?

Health-care staff, trained to standards of cleanliness, order and tidiness, may find the slovenliness of some patients intolerable. (In the same way, as community nurses may find offensive the behaviour of elderly people with what has been called the 'Diogenes syndrome'.) It is easy to rationalise the use of retraining measures for such patients on the grounds that it is necessary, for reasons of hygiene, to avoid fire hazards and to protect other patients' interests. Retraining patients to care for themselves and their environment may also ease the burden on the nursing staff and make the institutional management of such individuals easier and more pleasant. Each of these kinds of reason may carry some weight in justifying the use of behaviour modification techniques, but unless balanced by respect for the patient's rights and autonomy they can lead to abuse.

The use of aversion therapy in the treatment of some phobias and to help people — for example, to give up smoking, stop abusing drugs, or alcohol — can be justified reasonably easily in practice because the patient generally wants to overcome the phobia or dependence on addictive substances and, as a rule, can be consulted about treatment and can give informed and voluntary consent.

These cases are reasonably straightforward when the patient is competent to give consent. The case is much more complicated when the patient is mentally handicapped, mentally ill, senile or suffering the consequences of long-term institutionalisation. Here there may be serious doubts whether consent can be either informed or voluntary in any true sense. It becomes a matter of interpreting what the duty-to-care means in these circumstances for the health-care staff. They have to fall back on other kinds of justification: arguments that such measures are ultimately in the best interests of the patient (in the attempt to restore some degree of autonomy to the patient), or that the retraining is necessary to protect the rights (health and safety) of others, or that the staff cannot be expected to work in intolerable conditions (Ross 1981).

The argument that something is in the *best interests* of the patient is acceptable if, and only if, it is informed by a proper respect for the dignity of individual patients, by a concern to rehabilitate them, improve their quality of life, or at least to improve the general standards of patient care. Respect for the dignity of persons will obviously set limits to the degree or forms of coercion which are employed, and even the use of cigarettes as inducements may be ruled out on the grounds that they may damage the health of patients. There is always a risk that the assumption of fiduciary responsibility may lead to paternalism and even to abuse of patients if it is not limited by respect for persons. Studies of the extent of fire risk among mildly demented elderly people, for example, have shown that the risk is much less than it is imagined to be by neighbours and anxious professionals and that the use of alternative forms of heating can sometimes circumvent the need for institutionalisation. (Note 1)

It is far too easy for health professionals to rationalise their prejudices against people with different lifestyles or standards of cleanliness, and to impose a regimen on patients for their own convenience rather than the real benefit of patients. If this risk is recognised, then the use of behaviour modification techniques for the rehabilitation of those whose standards of self-care have deteriorated through illness or institutionalisation, may sometimes be justified on the kinds of grounds already discussed. The rights of nursing staff members to decent working conditions are important but not so important as to justify coercion of patients to conform to staff demands, when perhaps collective action by nurses may be required to ensure better staffing levels, modernisation of equipment and the provision of adequate resources.

Health education

Health education itself, in so far as it seeks to change people's attitudes and behaviour, raises ethical questions as well. Are nurses entitled to tell people that they should stop smoking, should not drink so much or that they should go on a diet? Or, more controversially, are nurses morally justified in advising people to practise contraception or to seek sterilisation? If so, how directive should this advice be? Should people just be given the facts and left to decide for themselves? Should nurses actively try to change people's attitudes and lifestyles? Should they be campaigning for legislation to control advertising of alcohol and tobacco? Should they support seat-belt legislation, drunk driving laws or compulsory fluoridation of water? Should they be involved directly in community development in areas of high unemployment and social deprivation? (GNC 1980, Coutts & Hardy 1985).

Health education, if it is to be relevant, must be related to the patterns of morbidity and mortality in society. In the past, the infectious diseases and diseases associated with poverty were responsible for high infant mortality rates and the deaths of young people. These diseases have been largely controlled by general improvements in the standard of living (better housing and diet), public health measures (better sewerage disposal, cleaner water supplies), and by medical measures (immunisation and the development of effective drugs). Today in the developed countries, the pattern of morbidity and mortality is quite different. Infant mortality rates have been dramatically reduced and most dying is done by the elderly. There has been a vast increase in the proportion of the population over the age of 50 years, and most illness in this group is lifestyle-related. Apart from accidental and violent deaths (a small proportion) the vast majority of deaths and morbidity in the population are associated with smoking, alcohol abuse, inappropriate diet and lack of exercise. While poverty and associated conditions of multiple deprivation are important factors, the epidemic of chronic and disabling diseases of middle and later life is clearly lifestyle-related. If the major causes of early death are to be eliminated, then people's attitudes and values have to be changed (McKeown 1976).

Obviously, the major ethical justification for health education is the same as that which was invoked to justify compulsory immunisation, notification of infectious diseases, and compulsory public health measures: namely, an appeal to the *common good*, on the basis of the principles of beneficence, justice to protect the rights (to health and safety) of the majority, even if it means restricting the rights of some individuals and dissenting minorities. (The issues of seat-belt legislation and fluoridation raise similar questions today.) The fact is, though, that legal and fiscal measures cannot be forced on a community entirely without their consent, even in a totalitarian state. Public opinion has to be informed and persuaded, a consensus created — and that is a task of health education. If health educationalists are not to give offence they have to respect the rights and autonomy of individuals, their right to decide on their own values and lifestyle. People cannot be forced to take responsibility for their health. They may be given inducements to do so, or subjected to various forms of sanctions if they do not do so.

If health education is to be effective, it may be necessary to use a wide variety of health education measures. It will not be sufficient just to give people the facts and leave them to make up their own minds, when millions of pounds are spent annually on advertising alcohol and tobacco. It will not be sufficient to promote the value of positive health through the education of individuals — children and adults — when these alternative attitudes and values are contradicted by the social circumstances in which they live. It will not be sufficient to try to influence health behaviour through taxation and legal measures when huge vested interests are at stake in the tobacco, alcohol and food industries. Advertising may need to be controlled, funds may have to be allocated for community development and the combating of social deprivation and poverty. State subsidies and tax incentives may need to be given to companies to diversify and phase out the production of things damaging health (Thompson 1987).

Health professionals have a fundamental responsibility to be health educators, in so far as their training as nurses, paramedical staff members or doctors must commit them to the promotion of health and not merely to the treatment of disease. The National Health Service was not intended as a national disease service. Health professionals have a responsibility for the *health* of their patients (Wilson 1975). The health professional therefore has a special responsibility to act as a role model. The nurse who is a heavy smoker or abuses alcohol cannot expect her advice to be taken seriously. Her credibility as a health professional is called in to question. This does not mean that all nurses have to be angels, but their example in taking responsibility for their own health is important. The high cigarette consumption among nurses as a profession may have many explanations, including the alternating periods of stress and boredom which characterises their work. However, the example of doctors in giving up smoking has not only had a dramatic effect on the incidence of heart disease and lung cancer in their ranks, but has obviously impressed their patients, who have given up smoking in large numbers (Coutts & Hardy 1985).

Health professionals, as a body of people with public responsibility for maintaining the health services, cannot simply rest content with passive implementation of health policies decided by other people. As those who see the casualties on the wards and in the community every day, they have a responsibility to try to use their political influence actively to shape health policies. Through their professional associations and unions, nurses have the power to influence public opinion and so achieve by political, legislative and fiscal means what cannot be achieved by individual counselling. However, respect for the rights of individuals must be maintained, when pressure is being exerted on individuals and nations to change their lifestyle. The ultimate justification for health education is that the rights of patients demand it — especially the right to know and the right to treatment.

Communication

Communication with patients is not only important as a means of discovering or conveying information, and as a means of expressing sympathy, encouragement and personal interest, it is also the single most important way of securing co-operation and compliance. In other words, communication plays a vital role in the management and control of patients (Fletcher 1971, Bennett 1976).

It has become fashionable to talk about the importance of communication in medicine and nursing, and to explain the failures in relationships with patients as being due to 'poor communication'. This explanation is misleading if it implies that health professionals are poor communicators. Experienced doctors and nurses are highly skilled at certain forms of directive managerial communication — using language and the selective disclosure of information as a means of securing patient compliance and as means of control. However, they may be much less skilled than their junior colleagues at listening to patients, communicating with patients as persons, understanding their personal needs, responding to their different levels of comprehension of information.

Research in health education shows up major problems in the attempts of health professionals to communicate with ordinary people, for several reasons: their use of specialist jargon, their different educational level and level of literacy, and their quite different life expectations (Baric 1982). Simple tests for readability and comprehensibility can now be applied to written material, such as patient information sheets and consent forms. It is both a professional and moral duty of nurses to ensure that patients can in fact read the information they are given, particularly when informed consent is required for treatment or participation in a clinical control trial (Church 1982).

Research into communication with patients in hospital, regarding their treatment or the likely effects of surgery, shows wide discrepancies between the levels of actual comprehension and recall by patients and that attributed to them by nurses, and doctors (in particular) (Ley 1976). The form of training to which health professionals are subjected, the demands of institutional life, and the need to 'manage' large number of patients, may make nurses and doctors less sensitive with the passage of time to the way manipulative communication can offend patients and create mistrust. (Patients often remark that they learn more from porters and cleaners than from medical and nursing staff. Nurses and doctors would do well to recognise that these hospital workers have an important role to play in communication with patients, and to consider why this is the case.)

First and foremost, all health professionals need to enlarge their repertoire of communication skills. In some circumstances 'controlling' and 'managerial' communication may be required and appropriate, particularly in a crisis, but the other more sensitive communication skills, associated with 'counselling' and 'helping' patients to sort out their own problems and take their own decisions, require quite different training and the development of quite different skills. On the whole, the traditional forms of education and training for health professions, as well as clinical experience, do not equip health professionals with these skills — if anything, the available evidence suggests that, in the process of their 'training' in patient care, there is 'serial desensitization' of nurses and doctors to the need for these skills (Bennett 1976).

Communication between nurses and patients can raise two kinds of ethical problems: first, when communication fails to express respect for the patient as a person; and, second, when the patient's right to know is ignored. The first kind of problem arises when hospital staff members talk over the heads of patients or, more seriously, fail to respect confidences. The power relationship between patient and health professional is an unequal one, and communication can be used to control the patient rather than to relate to him as a person. The sick or injured patient is often anxious and distressed because he does not understand what is happening to him or why it is happening. He is vulnerable and dependent. Not only does he need the reassurance which the expert can give him, but he needs information. The medical and nursing staff have a responsibility to share their knowledge and the specific information about the patient with him, and to share it in the most caring way.

7.3 Balancing the rights of patients with the interests of third parties

In general, and for very good reasons, the focus of training in nursing and medicine is on direct patient care, on the one-to-one relationship between carer and patient in the clinical situation. Less attention is given to the wider responsibilities in management, research and health promotion. Clinical practice is grounded on the more *individual*, or *'personalist'*, values of beneficence and respect for persons. The values on which the other functions of health care are based are the more *universal* values derivable from principles of justice.

In practice, nurses — like doctors and paramedical staff — usually have obligations to several patients at the same time. Because each nurse 'has only one pair of hands' and 'cannot be in two places at once', she has to make decisions about whom to give priority and how to do the best for all her patients. These more universal considerations of justice and the common good may suggest different responses to her than if she had only one patient to care for. The same could be said of doctors: the demands of teaching, administration, research and public health all introduce more universal obligations to be balanced against the rights of patients in the one-to-one clinical relationship.

Health professionals often feel most comfortable at the level of ethical decisions of a personal kind relating to individual patients and their health needs. Their expertise and clinical experience relate best to the treatment of individual patients and decisions about their management. A personalist ethic, based on 'caring', appears most appropriate to such situations. The doctor may well feel that his expertise (unless he is an epidemiologist and trained administrator) is not applicable to decisions about the general allocation of manpower and resources. Nurses on the other hand, while sharing the same personalist ethic, may have more experience in management of large groups of patients and feel less uneasy about making decisions based on the general good. The conflict between these different kinds of values, personalist and universal, come out most clearly where the rights of indi-vidual patients have to be balanced against the interests of third parties. The situations that may serve to illustrate some of the problems and dilemmas are: decisions to refuse the admission of a patient; persuading patients to 'volunteer' as research subjects in clinical trials and/or non-therapeutic research; the use of cases as teaching material; and decisions about allocation of resources.

Refusing to admit a patient

A classic dilemma facing a charge nurse may be whether she can accept responsibility for another patient when there is an acute shortage of staff and resources. The conflict here is between her straightforward duty to care for the patient who has been brought to the ward, and her duty to provide adequate care for the other patients on the ward (and perhaps to consider her staff, what it may be reasonable or unreason-able to expect of them in such a situation). An alternative way of viewing the problem is to see it as a conflict between the right to treatment of the patient seeking admission and the rights of those in the ward already receiving treatment. Either way there is a dilemma to be faced. Consider the following case:

Recently, when I was doing night duty as charge nurse in the acute admissions ward of the local psychiatric hospital, I was faced with a very painful decision. We were short of staff. This was due to the freeze on vacant posts — seemingly part of the policy of 'cuts' imposed by the local health authority; but also aggravated by an epidemic of 'flu which had affected several staff. We had been operating for several days below what I would regard as safe staffing levels. The duty doctor was a young trainee psychiatrist with little experience of the application of the Mental Health Act. However, we managed because we had most of the patients well under control and had not had a new admission for several days.

On the night in question, one of the patients on the ward, Mrs M, was upset by an accidental injury caused by another patient and became very disturbed and violent towards other patients and staff. I

called for help from the duty doctor, as I had only one staff nurse
and an auxiliary to deal with the demands of 10 disturbed patients.
We had difficulty subduing Mrs M and persuading her to take some
medication — a powerful tranquilliser — and were trying to calm
down the other patients, who had become very agitated, when we
were informed that the police were at Reception with a woman who
was hysterical, had attempted to slash her wrists and was being
abusive and violent towards the police. They were demanding that
she be admitted under the relevant section of the Mental Health Act
which gives police the authority to detain people who, in their
opinion, are mentally disordered.

The young doctor was undecided whether we could cope with the
new admission, but felt we ought to accept her because she was in a
bad way and needed immediate medical treatment. In the
circumstances I felt I had to refuse, as I knew we could not cope and
that the care of the other patients might be put at risk. The doctor
was angry, although he later admitted that he thought I was right to
refuse. The suicidal woman was given the necessary first aid and
some medication and taken to the police cells for the night, until
other arrangements could be made for her care.

In this case, the issues faced by the charge nurse concerned
the relative weight to be given to the rights of the various
patients in her care and the conflict between her responsibility to a whole ward of acutely ill patients and her duty to
help a particular woman who clearly needed urgent psychiatric attention.

At one level, the charge nurse's decision might appear
sensible and possibly the only thing to do in the circumstances. She did not perceive it as a moral dilemma in the
strict sense, but rather as a moral problem which she solved
by giving priority to the demands of justice to her staff and
the 10 patients on the ward. The young doctor clearly saw the
problem differently and gave greater weight to the needs of
the suicidal woman, perhaps because he felt responsible for
taking the legal decision to have her admitted on an Emergency Order and perhaps because he felt able to treat her
problem.

The tense and difficult situation gave it the proportions of
a 'crisis' for the overstretched staff, and this atmosphere of
crisis was aggravated by the differences between the charge
nurse and the doctor. In such circumstances it becomes
difficult to make sensible and responsible moral choices, and
the moral issues may in fact be secondary to other agendas
between the nursing and medical staff or hospital adminis-

tration. However, it is important to tease out what moral issues are involved and to develop models for sensible decision-making in such circumstances (see Chapter 9). Some of the most critical decisions faced by health care staff occur in situations where there are numerous people in need of urgent attention and limited staff and resources to deal with the emergency. Part of the problem again may relate to factors of a non-moral nature, such as the youth and inexperience of the doctor, or the sense of hopelessness of the charge nurse faced with staff shortages and an unsympathetic health authority, or the impotence of the whole team faced with 'the last straw' arrival of another patient.

The moral questions raised by this case are of various kinds. There are the questions which relate to the rights of the various patients involved, the apparent conflict between the rights of one and the rights of others. Clearly here no one patient's rights are absolute. As indicated in Chapter 6, rights are not absolute or unlimited. Provision of treatment or a bed, for one patient, for example, may mean that another patient is deprived or that there are less resources to go around for others. Sensible decisions have to be made in the best interests of all. In some cases this demand of justice may mean that a patient cannot be given treatment at a particular time, because all available resources are committed. Alternatively, in some situations of extreme emergency, where the life of a patient is at risk, less ill patients may have to suffer a degree of neglect for the sake of saving a life. In the one case the demands of the common good prevail, in the other case the right of a particular person to treatment. Both cases could be said to be requirements of the principle of justice, but in different circumstances. In theory we may derive most personal rights from the principle of respect for persons, but we may not be able to resolve conflicts of rights between different parties without other considerations based on justice and beneficence.

There are also questions raised by this case about the entitlement of nurses and doctors to administer compulsory treatment, with or without fulfilling the requirements and procedures of the Mental Health Act, for example, the administration of tranquillisers as a means of subduing a violent patient — whether or not the patient resists the treatment.

Some of these questions were covered in Chapter 5, when discussing the ambiguous status of the mentally disordered patient. Other questions raised by this type of case relate to the nurse's right to conscientious objection to assisting in treatments ordered by the doctor — a subject discussed in Chapter 3. Another area of concern, on which the Health Service trade union COHSE and the Royal College of Psychiatrists have pronounced, is the matter of the legal responsibility of staff in dealing with violent patients, both with respect to their own safety and in protecting themselves from subsequent litigation if charges of negligence or physical abuse are brought against staff (COHSE 1977, Royal College of Psychiatrists 1977). The issues here relate to the rights of the nurse or doctor, their own entitlement to justice — to fair conditions of service and protection from mischievous prosecution when coping with difficult and dangerous patients; and their duty of public accountability — in situations where the very legal powers and circumstances of compulsory detention of disturbed and vulnerable patients give rise to fears that patients may be abused or maltreated by staff. The provision of legal safeguards for the rights of psychiatric patients, in particular their rights of access to Mental Health Tribunal/Mental Welfare Commission in Britain, are necessary because of the peculiar powers exercised by health professionals under the law in the case of psychiatric patients, and the peculiar vulnerability of patients who are 'incompetent' by virtue of mental disorder.

Finally, there is a whole series of questions about the provision of adequate resources for psychiatric services. The low prestige of psychiatry and psychiatric nursing, and the low priority accorded to mental health services compared with the acute medical and surgical services, in spite of the large proportion of patients requiring psychiatric treatment and in spite of official recommendations to the contrary, raises questions about the rationality of health service planning and justice in health care generally. The kind of crisis which makes a charge nurse refuse to admit a patient demands more of the nurse than merely a gesture of non-cooperation. The wider 'political' responsibilities of nurses are painfully illustrated in such situations, and their protests may be the most successful way of drawing attention to the inadequacy of the service to these particularly vulnerable patients, who by and large are unable to defend their own rights to have proper care and treatment.

Persuading 'volunteer' research subjects

Nursing practice, like medical science, can only advance through properly controlled scientific research. The controls required are both scientific and ethical. Research which is not conducted according to proper scientific procedure is value-less, and research which is not conducted with proper respect for the rights of patients may become inhuman.

In order to be *scientific*, nursing research must be based on sound scientific knowledge and proper scientific methods. This means in the first instance that initial research must establish what has already been done in the field, to avoid unnecessary repetition of research and waste of public resources. It also means that the research instruments must be properly pre-tested to establish their validity, or well-tried methods should be used. The project must be based on sound research design, and undertaken by properly qualified research staff. These requirements are not only scientific but ethical. The researcher has an obligation in justice not to engage in research which is valueless and a waste of time and resources. This is not only because most research is funded from public money and involves the use of public resources, it is also to protect research subjects from unnecessary inves-tigations of no benefit to them or to anyone else.

In order to be *ethical*, nursing research must be based on prior assessment of risks and benefits of the research procedures. It would not be justified when the risks outweigh the benefits. If the research is of a clinical nature and carries potential risk, then prior laboratory tests and animal exper-iments are required out of respect for patients' rights and as an expression of the researcher's duty to care for her research subjects. Furthermore, the research would have to be based on the full informed and voluntary consent of the patient to participate in the research project, or, where the patient is not competent to give consent, special safeguards must be established to protect his rights (e.g. proxy consent or tribunals to monitor the research in the patient's interest) (WMA 1975, RCN 1977)

Clinical research may be therapeutic or non-therapeutic. Therapeutic research is directly related to the patient's complaint and the patient stands to benefit directly from the treatments or procedures used. Non-therapeutic nursing research is where patients participate in general investigations. For example, research aimed at improving patient care, techniques of management, nurse/patient communication, or general knowledge of the physiology or pathology of particular complaints, where the investigations are of a general nature and have neither any specific therapeutic purpose nor are of any direct benefit to the research subject. In practice, the distinction is not so clear-cut, for patients may stand to benefit in the long run from even the most academic studies of sociology or psychology, as they may from laboratory studies of the composition of the blood or the biochemistry of the brain. Furthermore, in randomised control trials using placebos, some patients may receive potentially therapeutic drugs or treatment and others no treatment at all.

However, in broad principle the distinction between therapeutic and non-therapeutic research is a useful one even if only to emphasise that the ethical safeguards in the latter type have to be more stringent. In general the risks taken in clinical research are justified on two grounds, first that there may be benefit for the patient and, secondly, that the research may contribute to the benefit of humanity even if it does not directly benefit the patient. The right of the patient to treatment includes the implicit assumption that they will co-operate in the trial of various procedures yet have the right to withdraw if they believe they are suffering harm.

It has been argued that the right of the patient to benefit from research carries with it a corresponding duty to assist in research which may be of benefit to other patients too. This duty is a moral duty which may or may not be recognised as such by the patient. It is not a duty which can be forced on anybody (McCormick 1976). The patient has a right to be properly informed and to give his consent without coercion. He also has a right to be informed of the risks and possible benefits, and to withdraw from any trial or research project without prejudice to his treatment.

The nurse or doctor in charge of patients in research trials has a special responsibility to protect the interests of the individual patients, to act as their advocate and to advise them about participation and withdrawal from experiments. Because patients in hospital are to some degree captive, it is important to ensure that they feel quite happy about partici- pation in a trial, particularly if it is not one from which they stand to benefit directly. However, staff members may also have to persuade patients to co-operate, and here the personal values of clinical practice and the more universal ones justifying research may come into conflict. These may be particularly acute in justifying clinical research involving children, prisoners, mentally disordered or mentally and physically handicapped people. In such cases, legal and insti- tutional safeguards are particularly important, to protect the wider interests of those not competent to give informed and voluntary consent — whether they stand to benefit or will merely be contributing to the welfare of others.

The issue of whether it is ethical to use children as subjects of clinical research has been hotly debated. On the one hand, it has been argued that children cannot be said to give consent that is either informed or voluntary in any proper sense. Children's lack of knowledge and understanding of the implications of medical procedures and even of the legal significance of consent may be said to invalidate any attempt to justify their use as research subjects on moral grounds. Children's dependency on adults for protection and advice makes them peculiarly vulnerable to moral pressures, and it is doubtful whether their consent could really be voluntary (Ramsey 1976, 1977). On the other hand, it has been argued that this issue cannot be settled by arguments based alone on the *rights* of the individual (child), for advances in the treat- ment of paediatric disorders often cannot be made without research or clinical trials involving children.

Again, it can be argued that the right to benefit from new discoveries in the clinical sciences carries with it the corre- sponding moral duty to contribute to the advance of clinical research, and this correspondence between rights and duties applies to children as much as to anyone else. This argument was advanced by McCormick (1976) and in the Belmont Report (DHEW 1978). However, in both sources it is emphasised that the researcher has a fundamental duty to protect the rights of children and incompetent adults, to prevent their exploitation. Furthermore, the researcher has an obligation to avoid subjecting human subjects to hazardous procedures, where other procedures involving competent adults or animals as subjects would do just as well, or where the risk outweighs the possible benefits.

Those people who are contemplating research involving children (or mentally disordered individuals) sometimes fall back on the consent of the parents or a relative. This can be an attempt to safeguard the interests of vulnerable individuals, but the question can be raised too whether the insistence on proxy consent is not more to protect the doctor or institution from legal action. Ramsey (1976, 1977) maintained that it is never permissible to use children as research subjects in non-therapeutic research, and that proxy consent does not make it ethical either. McCormick (1974) argued, on the other hand, that since the ultimate justification for clinical research is that it contributes to the common good, and justice requires that we are prepared to accept risks ourselves if we wish to benefit from medical discoveries (either in the short term or the long term), then we ought to be able to understand the principle of this exchange if we have the capacity. Even if we do not have the capacity it can be argued by analogy that we would give our consent if we could understand, and should therefore not be deprived of the right to contribute to the common good merely because we are not competent to give fully informed and voluntary consent. In fact, it can be doubted whether even the consent of normal adult patients can ever be fully informed or completely voluntary, and with children it is just a difference of degree. This is a highly controversial area in the ethics of clinical research, and while more often than not doctors have to take the key decisions, nevertheless nurses may have to cope with the enquiries of both children and their parents, and will therefore be required to have a clear view on where they stand on these issues — especially if they have to seek the 'consent' of the child.

In reality, the health professional has to exercise discretion about how much to tell and to judge whether consent is being given under duress. Respect for persons and the duty to care stand in a relationship of tension to one another. A degree of beneficent paternalism is necessary to interpret the needs of the individual, to judge his competence, to decide what is in his best interests. But paternalism can become officious and arrogantly indifferent to individuals if it is not based on respect for persons and their rights.

The establishment of Ethics of Research Committees in Britain (Institutional Review Boards in the United States) has been a major step forward in the attempt to monitor research involving human subjects. This came about in the first instance as the result of public concern over the possible abuse of patients as 'human guinea pigs' and, more seriously, the abuse of captive subjects such as prisoners and the mentally ill in research not only for clinical purposes but for merely commercial ends (Pappworth 1967, DHEW 1978). Researchers are required to submit research protocols for scrutiny by these committees, to ensure that they fulfil the requirements of sound scientific and ethical research. In some cases these committees may insist on direct monitoring of the ongoing research, or may require periodic reports to ensure that the general guidelines are being adhered to by all concerned. Nurses are increasingly taking a place on these interprofessional and multidisciplinary committees. In this role they have important professional and moral responsi- bilities, not only to ensure the proper vetting of nursing research but to provide a considered nursing viewpoint on the implications of the research proposed on patient care and well-being, as well as the implications for staffing and resources. Nurses, also arguably, have a responsibility to ensure that Ethics of Research Committees actually work and do their business in a conscientious way. Surveys of some such committees suggest that there is a lot of room for improvement (Thompson et al 1981, Goldman 1982).

Use of patients as teaching material

Should patients be used as teaching material for the training of doctors and nurses? Should patients with rare disorders or unusual complications be expected to put up with the additional inconvenience, embarrassment and even discomfort of being examined by students? In a major teaching centre, where the population does not have the opportunity of being treated in non-teaching hospitals, should patients be given the choice of consent or refusal to act as demonstration material for clinical tutorials? And what about the right to privacy of psychiatric patients and the dying?

Clinical training without the opportunity to work on real patients would be like learning to swim on dry land. Here the justification for compromising the right to privacy of individual patients is that the patient stands to benefit by having highly trained staff to care for him. Alternatively, the common good of all patients is served by having properly trained staff. However, this does not give medical or nursing instructors an unlimited right to do as they like with patients.

The requirements for the provision of sound clinical training for nurses (like the demands of medical research, health-care planning and public health measures) are such that they tend to give greater importance to considerations of the common good than to the specific needs or interests of individual patients. The nurse on the ward or the junior medical resident with a particular interest in and clinical responsibility for the individual patient may feel protective towards 'their' patients and critical of the insensitivity of those passing through on a teaching round. This tension between universal and personal values in health-care is well illustrated here. Neither view is exclusively right. Each needs to be tempered by the other. Institutionalised health care imposes some limitations on personal rights, including the right to privacy, but teaching and research institutions and hospitals generally need to be humanised as well.

Justice demands that patients with unusual and 'exotic' disorders should not be unduly exposed to students, with or without their consent. Even unconscious patients deserve to have their privacy respected and dignity protected. Lack of respect tends to breed insensitivity, callousness and lack of consideration in trainees. Some patients may be at risk of being over-researched, over-investigated, over-scrutinised because they are 'interesting teaching material'. Some reasonable and just limits have to be set to the demands made on such patients. The duty of patients to contribute to the common good by participating in clinical teaching is not unlimited. Apart from the need to preserve the trust and goodwill of patients by not exploiting them or trying their patience beyond endurance, professionals also have a duty to protect the dignity and privacy of those in their care. This is particularly important if the complaint makes them vulnerable (as in cases of mental illness) or liable to embarrassment (as in cases of pregnancy, disfiguring injury and handicap, or venereal disease).

It may be questioned whether something that places additional stress on anxious and distressed patients (e.g. disturbed psychiatric patients), such as exposure to a group of students, is morally justified even with the patient's 'consent'. The tutor may have to decide against using particular patients, however interesting, because of their vulnerability — that is his/her professional responsibility. On the other hand, it needs to be stressed that the expectations of people with regard to their privacy vary according to their situation. People tend to expect the greatest degree of privacy and strictest confidentiality to be observed when they are visited in their own homes or see health professionals in a private consultation. However, when people enter public institutions they recognise the implicit restrictions on their rights and are often explicitly obliged to surrender some degree of their privacy. In an institutional setting the health professionals may be more anxious about privacy and confidentiality than patients are (where much intimate information about patients may be common knowledge on the ward). Nevertheless, professionals cannot ignore the need of individuals for privacy, and they have a primary moral duty to protect the rights of the patients entrusted to their care.

Allocation of resources

Although the dilemmas of resource allocation in health care are discussed more fully in the next chapter, there are some features of these dilemmas which arise here while we are looking at questions where the rights of individuals have to be balanced against the interests of third parties. Let us consider a few examples. Should elderly patients be discharged from hospital to make way for more acute cases if there is a doubt that they will be able to cope on their own, even with domiciliary services and support? Should nursing staff be allocated according to need or according to the number of patients? Should more effort be put into nursing those who might show real improvement, or should all patients get equal treatment even if their state is chronic? How are decisions to be taken to allocate drugs and medical equipment where these are in short supply?

In real life, decisions *have* to be taken and these may be both painful and subsequently found to be mistaken or based on inadequate knowledge. All decisions where the rights of one patient have to be balanced against those of other patients or third parties may involve agonising choices. In formal terms it may be a choice between the demands of personal care or the individual patient and justice for a larger group of patients or society. In practical terms, it may be a matter of responding to external pressures and the internal guilt and anxiety generated by an unresolvable tension between conflicting duties. The extreme case may be a medical emergency such as an air crash or train disaster in which many people are injured or dying and there are limited medical supplies and perhaps only one qualified doctor or nurse available. As in similar situations in wartime, the responsible health professional may have to adopt a policy of *triage* — dividing the victims into three groups: those who must be left to die because they are beyond help, those who can wait for treatment later, and those who must be attended to first because they need treatment urgently and stand to benefit from it most. (How do we reconcile the conflicting demands of the principles of beneficence, justice and respect for persons here?)

Faced with several patients with chronic renal failure — with that is, similar pathology and urgent need, and with only one dialysis machine — who is to be given priority? Generally, the decision will be the doctor's, but if there are no obvious clinical criteria which would decide the issue in favour of one patient rather than another, other criteria might have to be considered, and nurses might get drawn into discussion of the available options. Would the decision be made most fairly by drawing lots or by adhering to a first-come-first-served basis? Would attempts to assess the usefulness/value/importance of individuals be reasonable or invidious? Attempts to involve patients in group decisions about the allocation of a dialysis machine would seem to be unfair. In such circumstances, decision by team consensus or by outside assessors might be justified if there were objective grounds on which the choice might be made. However, the judgements would tend in practice to be based either on the assessment of probabilities on the basis of personal experience or the subjective judgement of professionals. In the case of a real moral dilemma, where there are no practical strategies to avoid the problem of choice, the responsible health professionals have to be prepared to take a decision and to live with the guilt and anxiety which that responsibility entails. (It has been remarked that doctors are paid well 'to pad their shoulders' to carry the burden of responsibility. Perhaps the difficulty experienced by the nurse is that, faced with the similar clinical responsibility in some situations, she does not have the padding.)

In making decisions affecting the lives and well-being of individuals in their care, health professionals act as guardians and advocates of the rights of their patients. They have to make decisions based on their knowledge, expertise and available resources. They will have to exercise courageous initiative and be willing to take risks as they try to effect the best compromise between the demands of justice, beneficence and respect for the rights of individual patients.

Patients' rights and the responsibilities of health professionals have to be considered in the context of the rights of the rest of society — for all members of the public are potential patients, including all the staff who work in the health services. Because all of us are potential patients (including doctors and nurses) we all must have an interest in protecting patients' rights. The right to know, the right to privacy and the right to treatment are all better understood by health professionals who have experienced the impotence and vulnerability of patienthood. Health professionals who take their duties seriously will also be willing to act as advocates defending the rights and dignity of patients. They will also be aware that as public officers they have a responsibility to uphold the common good and to promote the health of the whole community.

NOTES AND REFERENCES

1 Research by the Department of Geriatric Medicine at the University of Edinburgh does not support the common view that demented people living at home constitute a serious fire risk to themselves and others. On the contrary, available evidence from the Chief Fire Officer for Lothian and Borders, points to most domestic fires being associated with alcohol abuse; and, over a period of 10 years up to 1982, not a single fire in the Region occurred in houses or flats occupied by patients known to the psychiatric services as demented.

Baric L 1982 Measuring family competence in the health maintenance and health education of children. WHO, Copenhagen

Bennett A E (ed) 1976 Communication between doctors and patients. Nuffield Provincial Hospitals Trust, London, Ch 2

Church M 1982 How do they read you? Edinburgh, Scottish Health Education Group.

Clark B 1978 Whose life is it anyway? Amber Lane Press, Oxford

COHSE 1977 The management of violent or potentially violent patients. Confederation of Health Service Employees, London

Coutts L C, Hardy L K 1985 Teaching for health: The nurse as a health educator. Churchill Livingstone, Edinburgh

Fletcher C M 1971 Communication in medicine. Nuffield Provincial Hospitals Trust, London

Goldman J 1982 Inconsistency and institutional review boards. JAMA 248 (2), 197–202

GNC 1980 Guidelines on health education. General Nursing Council for Scotland, Edinburgh

Ley P 1976 Towards better doctor–patient communication. In: Bennett A E (ed) Communication between doctors and patients. Oxford University Press, Oxford

McCormick R 1974 Proxy consent in the experimental situation. Perspectives in biology and medicine 18, 2–20

McCormick R 1976 Experiments in children: Sharing in sociality. Hastings Centre Report no. 6, 41–46

McKeown T 1976 The role of medicine. Nuffield Provincial Hospitals Trust, London

Pappworth M H 1967 Human guinea pigs: Experimentation in man. Routledge & Kegan Paul, London

Ramsey P 1976 The enforcement of morals: non-therapeutic research on children. Hastings Centre Report no. 6, 21–39

Ramsey P 1977 Children as research subjects: A reply. Hasting Centre Report no. 7, 40–42

RCN 1977 Ethics related to research in nursing. Royal College of Nursing, London

Royal College of Psychiatrists 1977 Guidelines on the care and treatment of mentally disturbed offenders. British Journal of Psychiatry Bulletin, April

Ross T 1981 Thought control. Nursing Mirror, April 23. (See also other articles on psychiatric ethics in the same series)

Thompson I E 1976 Suicide and philosophy. Contact 54(3), 9–23

Thompson I E 1987 Personal rights and public policy: Dilemmas in health education and prevention. In: Proceedings of the Twelfth World Conference on Health Education. International Union for Health Education, Health Education Bureau,

Thompson I E et al 1981 Research ethical committees in Scotland. British Medical Journal 282, 718–720

UKCC 1984 Code of Professional Conduct for the Nurse, Midwife and Health Visitor. United Kingdom Central Council for Nursing, Midwifery and Health Visiting, London

DHEW 1978 Protection of human subjects of biomedical and behavioral research. Federal Register 43 (53). US Departments of Health, Education and Welfare, Washington DC

Wilson M 1975 Health is for people. Darton, Longman and Todd, London

WMA 1975 Declaration of Helsinki. World Medical Association, New York. (Reprinted in: Duncan A S et al (eds) (1977/81) Dictionary of medical ethics)

8

Nurses and society

8.1 Conflicts between the professional and political duties of the nurse

The two previous chapters attempted to clarify some of the moral issues which arise in direct nurse–patient encounters without examining the broader issues of the nurse's administrative and public responsibilities. Attention was confined to moral dilemmas in interpersonal relationships between nurses and their patients in order to bring out the nature of patients' *rights* and the professional *duties* of nurses. In so doing we have skirted round the larger issues of social justice in health care, but could not avoid mentioning them altogether. This is because the interpersonal moral questions in nursing arise within a broader social context and the answers to questions about patients' rights and the duties of nurses depend on broader principles and beliefs about the role of nurses in society and the nature of the National Health Service.

Chapter 4 began with the assertion that ethics is concerned in a fundamental way with power and power sharing. This connection between ethics and power relationships was affirmed in order to challenge the popular view of professional ethics, which can be expressed as a series of interconnected beliefs as follows: that ethics is just about caring for people; that caring is about feelings; that feelings are personal and subjective; and, therefore, that ethics is a matter of personal and subjective judgement.

Of course, caring is of fundamental importance in human relationships. No one could deny this. However, caring can be patronising, caring can be sentimental, caring can be selective. For care without proper recognition of the individual's objective needs and right to preserve their independence can be intrusive and unwanted or dependency-inducing. The person who needs help wants competent help to deal with their problem. They are not necessarily looking for 'a meaningful relationship'.

Caring cannot be simply a matter of feeling or sentiment if it is to be an adequate basis of ethics in general or of nursing ethics in particular. The concept of 'care' in Judeo–Christian thought has more practical origins. 'Caritas' in the Latin tradition, or 'agape' in Greek, are not primarily concerned with how you *feel* about someone, but with how you *deal* with someone. Caring for someone means that you act for their good, assist them to achieve their goals in life and fulfilment. In theological language, the ultimate goal of caritas or agape is the salvation of the other person, and the word 'salvation' means 'to be made whole'. In that sense, the goal of caring is always to help others to achieve their optimum fulfilment as human beings. For the person who has been injured (and are we not all injured in some way or other?), the need is for healing, to be made whole. For the person who is sick, the need is to be restored to health. Patients need to be 'put back on their feet', to recover their independence (where possible), to feel that they are in control of their lives again.

Obviously, we are all vulnerable, and we may even be afflicted by the same problems as the patients we care for. This is not necessarily a bad thing. In fact, the experience of suffering may not only make us more sympathetic (from Latin *sum* with, *patior* to suffer) but it may also help us to empathise with our patients, that is, view the world as they see it, from the inside. Furthermore, the factors which attract us into nursing and other caring professions may be determined by our own unconscious agendas, our own need for help, our own fear of illness or death (Feifel 1967). Psychological studies of the helping personality show that personal experiences in childhood, or suffering and bereavement in adolescence, may be powerful motivators in the type of person attracted to 'caring' for other people. However, if the choice of nursing or medicine is just an unconscious form of autotherapy, simply a means of trying to deal with our own problems or anxieties, then 'patients' will suffer as we work out our own agendas, or 'act out' our own 'scripts' (Eadie 1975).

'Caring' can be dangerous if we do not understand its true dynamics, that is, the complex psychological forces which come into operation when we are in the powerful position of 'helpers', relative to weak and dependent 'patients' or 'clients'. This is why psychiatrists in training and psychiatric nurses are encouraged to undergo personal psychoanalysis, or to participate in group therapy, as this process obliges the carer to explore his or her deeper feelings and often hidden ulterior motives. While the care and attention of a good nurse can 'do one a power of good', officious, intrusive or over-bearing and patronising 'care', like the corresponding forms of bad parenting, can be very destructive too.

Preceding chapters have explored the moral implications of the complex dynamics of nurse–patient relationships and the responsibilities within such relationships. If we remember that the term 'dynamics' means power (from Greek *dynamis*, power), then we may understand that in such expressions as interpersonal dynamics, group dynamics, psychodynamics we are actually dealing with different kinds of power relation-ships and forms of power sharing. Nurses may not have too much difficulty accepting that ethics has to do with power and power sharing in these senses, particularly in interpersonal relationships. However, they appear to have more difficulty in accepting that ethics also covers issues of power and power sharing, in teaching, in management and administration, in research and health education, and in politics and economics in the wider sense as well — both in lobbying for resources within the National Health Service, and in the politics of health in national politics. If nurses really care about the well-being of their patients and are not merely caring for patients, they soon discover that ethics and politics are continuous with one another, that caring and sharing, respect for persons and justice, values and power relationships are all interconnected.

There appear to be two reasons why nurses have difficulty seeing the connection. The first has to do with the altruistic values on which nursing has been traditionally based. These values of 'caring', 'selfless devotion', 'self-sacrifice', are all important, and many nurses set a remarkable example of living up to these idealistic standards. However, it is easy to caricature the nurse as a kind of other-worldy 'angel', because the professing of these values without a balancing emphasis on justice and respect for her own needs can lead either to the nurse 'making a martyr of herself' or to a kind of hypocrisy about the nurse's natural concern with power, status and even money. Altruism, what is sometimes referred to as 'cold charity', lacks genuineness and warmth because the philanthropist does not care for himself very much.

The second reason has to do with the ambivalent attitudes in middle class society to politics and money. In his analysis of the origins of capitalism, in *The Protestant Era*, Paul Tillich discusses these ambivalences in the 'Protestant work ethic': on the one hand, railing against 'serving God and Mammon', or 'grubbing for filthy lucre', and meddling in 'dirty politics'; and on the other hand espousing the values of financial thrift, honest work to earn a living, and striving to realise the 'Kingdom of God' or an ideal 'theocratic Utopia' on earth. (Tillich, 1957).

At one level there appears to be an obvious conflict between the values of the kind of altruism based on a subjective understanding of 'caring' and the demands of getting involved in trade union activity or becoming directly involved in local or national politics, or between the idealistic picture of the nurse as 'pure as the driven snow' and being prepared to be 'contaminated by the world' of 'money grubbing' and 'dirty politics'.

The remainder of this chapter will consider a number of issues which bear on the political responsibilities of the nurse, issues where the personal values of caring come into abrasive contact with the realities of power: within the nursing hierarchy, between nurses and other professionals, between different departments in the competition for limited staff or resources, between different professional groups in the struggle to achieve advantageous outcomes for themselves in negotiations over pay and working conditions, and between vested commercial and political interests which determine the proportion of national resources allocated by the Government to the Health Service, compared with, say, Social Services, Education, or Defence.

Nurse tutors do their students a disservice if they do not address these real-life issues in nursing. If the only values professed are those based on a personalist ethic of caring, then the nurses produced will be ill-prepared to deal with the harsh economic and political realities of nursing. It will be a training for frustration without the basic skills to handle the 'nitty gritty' details of what caring means in terms of pounds and pence. Ethics in our terms means among other things that nurses themselves must have enough influence to command respect in 'the corridors of power', when it comes to decision-making about resources and health policy.

8.2 Withdrawal of labour, or the 'right' of nurses to strike

Strikes and various forms of so-called 'industrial action' have become commonplace among the health-care workers. A variety of forms of industrial action has been taken by hospital porters and ancillary staff and paramedical staff. In 1979 junior hospital doctors went on strike for better pay and working conditions. Nurses traditionally have been reluctant to take strike action, although they have staged demonstrations. A 'work-to-rule' by nurses at a major psychiatric hospital in Scotland by way of protest at 'unacceptable cuts in staff, which put both patients and staff at risk' was clearly motivated by concern about standards of patient care and their own working conditions. Are nurses ever justified in taking industrial action, working to rule or going on strike? The various trade unions representing nurses in Britain have different policies on this issue. Even if nurses do not go on strike, what attitude should they adopt towards other health-service workers engaged in industrial disputes?

Traditionally, the Royal College of Nursing has adopted a policy opposed to nurses taking industrial action, particularly in pursuit of wage claims, and has favoured 'no strike' wage deals with nurses, based on guarantees from the Government that would underwrite the review, and arbitration over wages affecting nurses, for example, by having them index-linked to the rate of inflation or comparability with other professions such as the Civil Service. During the 1987 National Conference of the Royal College of Nursing, this policy was changed in favour of qualified support for nurses taking industrial action in circumstances where standards of patient care and staff morale are so badly affected that the health and well-being of both are put at risk.

The Code of Professional Conduct unequivocally rejects strike action as a legitimate weapon to be used by nurses, particularly if such action puts at risk the safety of patients (RCN 1977, clause 4).

At the time of the publication of the RCN Code a group of nursing students commented as follows:

> On the subject of industrial action most students think that they have a duty to ensure the safety of patients when colleagues or other health care workers withdraw their labour. A few thought that it might be necessary to withdraw their labour in extreme situations when improvements in standards of care are denied by employing authorities. This action would only be contemplated in extreme situations and only in units when patients' lives would not be at risk, for example in day hospitals. (RCN 1977)

Other critics have echoed this view more strongly, namely that nurses as public officers charged with the care of patients have a duty to protect and if necessary to take industrial action when the standards of available patient care fall below acceptable levels and endanger the health and safety of patients. This point was made forcefully in the wake of the enquiry into the conditions at the Normansfield Mental Hospital (HMSO 1978). Here the enquiry found that the appalling standards of patient care were partly attributable to the intolerance and high-handedness of the responsible consultant, and also to the poor state of buildings and equipment, poor staffing levels and poor morale. Whether demoralised nurses in such a hospital could have organised effective industrial action may be doubted, but considerations of justice demanded that some drastic action should have been taken, that in the interests of the long-term safety and well-being of the patients the risk of short-term inconvenience to patients should have been accepted.

More radical criticism has been that if other industrial workers have the right to strike, then nurses, as employees of the largest single 'industry' in Europe, also have the right to withdraw their labour if negotiations with their employers over pay and working conditions have reached an impasse and there is no other way of achieving settlement. These critics have argued that the non-striking posture of nurses lays them open to exploitation by the employing authority — a risk which is especially great in a huge nationalised industry like the NHS, where decisions about the allocation of resources are taken by bureaucrats or politicians in Whitehall, far removed from the actual working conditions of nurses. Furthermore, it is impossible to separate issues of patient care from the pay and working conditions of health-care staff, since poor staffing levels and poor working conditions affect staff morale and the standards of patient care tend to fall. The idealism and dedication of nurses makes them vulnerable to moral blackmail in pay negotiations, and their compliance only delays the necessary improvements to outmoded services and dilapidated buildings.

How do we sort out the moral imperatives? The RCN Code gives ultimate priority to the principle of beneficence, or the duty to care, when discussing the nurse's obligations. In a sense, this is the easy, more respectable and least controversial line to take. It is in accord with the model of the nurse unselfishly sacrificing herself in the service of humanity. However, beneficence alone does not define moral duty, as it does not take account of the rights of others nor of the requirements of justice either to nurses or to their patients.

The principle of respect for persons requires that the nurse recognises the patient's rights, including the right to adequate treatment. Where treatment is below standard to the point of endangering the health or even the life of the patient, the nurse has a duty to do something about it; this overrides her duty merely to continue to perform her prescribed institutional duties. The patient's right to privacy and respect for his dignity is compromised in overcrowded, poorly staffed hospitals; and the right to know is violated if patients are kept in ignorance of the fact that they could expect a better standard of care. The principle of respect for persons also applies to the nurse herself: she is entitled to decent working conditions and a fair wage — within the limits of available resources; and she is entitled to protect herself against being unjustly exploited. What this means in specific situations would have to be examined. The form of protest or strike action taken would have to be proportionate to the degree of risk to patients if action were not taken, and to the degree of exploitation or intimidation suffered by nurses.

The principle of justice might also take precedence over the principle of beneficence in specific circumstances where patients suffer gross injustice, owing to inadequate staff or medical resources which put them at risk, or where health-care staff suffer gross injustice which threatens their well-being and standards of patient care. Again the action taken, if it were to be morally justifiable, would have to be proportional to the risk suffered by patients or the injustice suffered by health-care staff. Here it is easy to exaggerate, and the rhetoric of pay negotiations, for example (especially when they are conducted before the media), invariably exaggerates the 'risks' and 'injustice' involved. It is relatively easy to envisage the kind of extreme situations where strike action would not only be justified but becomes a moral duty. If nurses were terrorised and threatened with loss of their jobs and banishment if they did not do their duty, even though paid only starvation wages, then they would be justified in staging a revolt. However, in less dramatic circumstances it is often more difficult to determine whether the nurse's duty to care should take priority or whether nurses should withdraw their labour in pursuance of justice and proper respect for their rights and those of their patients.

On the matter of strikes, the law in the UK is rather confused. Discussing strikes and the NHS, Gerald Dworkin observed that in terms of section 5 of the Conspiracy and Protection of Property Act of 1875, 'It is a criminal offence for any health service employee wilfully and maliciously to break a contract where there is a risk to a patient's life or limb.' However he went on to point out that industrial action within the NHS has in some instances attempted to remain technically within the law by adopting two strategies: (a) work-to-rule or work-to-contract, so that the letter if not the spirit of the contract is honoured, and (b) by undertaking to deal with 'emergencies' so that those who are at risk are not affected by action taken (Dworkin 1977).

The risk in such strategies is that they become hypocritical.

The work-to-contract is in reality a strike with serious implications for many patients — in terms of unfair delays, deterioration in standards of care, or worse. The 'emergencies
only' policy is a farce, when porters or ambulancemen decide
which cases are emergencies. Even doctors cannot in good
faith justify a policy of selective action that is designed to
affect administration rather than clinical care. As Lord
Amulree said in a House of Lords debate: 'The decision to
treat emergencies is . . . humbug, because one cannot tell
what is an emergency' (RCN 1977).

It is part of the rhetoric of industrial disputes to talk glibly
about 'the right to strike'. There is no such right in law where
there is risk to the health and safety of other people, and a
strike is even less acceptable in moral terms if it puts others
at risk. The fact is that the talk is loudly about 'rights' when
we wish to draw attention to injustice or felt justice of our
cause, but rights cannot be rights if they are exercised at the
price of harm to others. Here the considerations of formal
justice have to be tempered by respect for persons and the
duty to care for others. The alleged 'right to strike' is not
enforceable in law; on the contrary, it often means using
extra-legal means to bring pressure on employers or the state
to yield to demands.

The concern was expressed in the 1970s, for example, by
Professor Kahn Freund, that instead of trade unions being the
victims of a repressive system of legislation which discrimi-
nates against them, 'The danger has shifted. It seems that
there is a spreading belief that the law cannot put any limits
on any action taken in the course of an industrial dispute'
(Journal of Medical Ethics 1977). His argument was that if any
kind of industrial action for whatever cause, however trivial,
justifies extra-legal action, then there is a serious risk that the
law and legal institutions will be brought into disrepute and
society will be thrown into anarchy. On the other hand, there
are those who would argue that such revolutionary action is
necessary, because the structure of contemporary society is
inimical to the health of people and the health services are
in a state of collapse. However, the majority of people would
not agree and would certainly not consider that such extreme
measures are justified to achieve the necessary reform and
improvements in society. The measures taken by many

governments to restrict the power of trade unions are taken on the strength of such views, or their ability to put across to voters the fear that trade unions are either in the business of pursuing selfish ends or anarchic political action. The risk is that if such action is taken too far and the power of organised labour is undermined to the degree that workers have no real power or legitimate mechanisms to negotiate over pay or working conditions, then the situation is ripe for riot and anarchy. A nice balance has to be maintained between the power of governments, employers and workers if the demands of justice and the common good are to be properly safeguarded.

From a moral point of view, while nurses may be justified in taking strike action if, and only if, there is serious deterioration of services and risk to the lives of patients, it is more difficult to establish a credible case based on arguments that poor wages for nurses threaten the health of patients. The danger is that the use of the rhetoric of 'campaigning for better standards of patient care' tends to be heard by politicians and the general public as special pleading, and is often regarded with scepticism by those commanding the control of resources. It may well be not only more honest, but more telling to separate the issues of standards of care from disputes about wage claims. Each issue can be the basis of responsible protest (or even strike action) in appropriate circumstances.

The moral issue about strike action by nurses turns to some extent on the status of nurses. Traditionally, the caring and consulting professions have been characterised by a self-professed altruism — 'selfless service on behalf of others'. A leading member of the legal profession has described his profession, without apparent irony, as one of the caring professions. Those who aspire to the status of 'professionals' have to persuade the public that they are a responsible and trustworthy body of people. This is why one of the first steps in seeking recognition and formal statutory registration as a profession is often to formulate a code of ethics (Freidson 1970). The difficulty with this stand is that it seems to be incompatible with the values on which other industrial and public utility workers base their claims to take strike action in pursuance of just settlements of their grievances. The demands for some degree of professional autonomy, respect for nursing knowledge and expertise, recognised status and appropriate financial reward depend upon nurses fulfilling the other criteria the public expects of caring professionals — objectivity, non-discrimination in the treatment of clients, altruism and dedication to duty, and commitment to care (often over and beyond the call of duty). These values are often incompatible, and are seen to be incompatible, with strategies of industrial action. In a sense, nurses may have to choose between being regarded as professionals and enjoying the ambiguous privileges of that status or accepting the status of health service workers along with the rest and being subject to the same kinds of employment legislation and negotiating rights, including the right to strike, as other workers and public servants.

The difficulty facing both doctors and nurses in a nationalised health service is that it is difficult for them to act as autonomous or self-employed professionals might. The greater equality in the distribution of health care which the nationalised system of health care in Britain was supposed to achieve (and has to some extent achieved) (DHSS 1980) was brought about, among other things, by health professionals sacrificing some of their privileges and autonomy. This was supposed to correct a situation where doctors and other specialists might profit from the nation's ill-health. Today the moves to reintroduce private medicine in the health service are, it is claimed, to allow a greater degree of choice to the public. The argument gives the right to choose and individual autonomy, for those who can afford it, higher priority than considerations of equality of opportunity, access and outcome for all groups in society. Part of the argument is based on the escalating cost of health services, and the need to make these profitable where possible, to finance care to others. Whether the profit motive and the provision of good health services and social services to all citizens are compatible is a matter of the greatest moment in the debate about the ethics and politics of health care.

However, there is considerable confusion in the debate about the 'right' to strike, when applied to health service workers, and whether in a nationalised system of health care or a profit-making private sector the problems are essentially the same. These industrial relations problems require urgent attention, and in particular there is a need for better nego-tiation and conciliation efforts to deal with the pay and working conditions of health workers. Changes will only be brought about by pressure from the nursing unions. The unionisation of nursing labour has many advantages. It gives considerable power to nurses, but it is a power which has to be seen to be used responsibly, within the limits of professional morality, if nurses are to command the respect of society and society's attention to the justice of their cause.

8.3 Dilemmas of resource allocation in health care

Headlines like the following highlight the problems facing health-care staff: 'COSTS "KILLING" KIDNEY CHILDREN: LACK OF MONEY AND DONORS DENY THE YOUNG VITAL TREATMENT' (The Guardian, Jan 15, 1982).

'Funds for kidney units are running seriously short. About half the 2200 people whose kidneys fail, die because there are no facilities to save them,' Professor Cyril Chantler of Guy's Hospital said yesterday. 'Most are over 45, but only 61 children under 15 were treated in 1980, while an estimated 90 suffered fatal kidney failure.'
'If there was enough money to treat every kidney failure, we would be treating 1000 more patients a year and would save hundreds of lives. It costs £10 000 a year to keep someone on a kidney machine. A transplant costs £5,000 a year for five years. So prevention not only saves lives, it makes economic sense,' said Professor Chantler.
'Britain is sixteenth in the European league for kidney treatment. The Swiss do more, and both Spain and Cyprus treat more patients per head of population.'

Similarly, emotive reports have dramatically highlighted the life-saving character of heart transplant surgery, in spite of the high failure rate and poor survival rate of these costly and still experimental procedures. Dr Peter Draper (Unit for the Study of Health Policy, Guy's Hospital, London) has argued that the money spent on heart transplant surgery would perhaps be better spent on health education, since most of the heart conditions being treated by transplant surgery are prevent-able (Draper & Popay 1980).

Two more controversial examples illustrate rather different problems: first, the justifiability of assisting couples otherwise unable to have children to have a child by *in vitro* fertilisation, and, second, the justifiability of life-saving surgery and long-term intensive care for seriously defective newborns.

These cases may not fall within the area where nurses have much power to influence decision-making, but they are important because they raise general questions of resource allocation dilemmas for nurses, and because issues of resource allocation are matters of general public interest and health policy and not the exclusive preserve of doctors or any particular class of professional. In fact, the judgement of doctors in these matters may be questioned because they often have a vested interest in defending the prestige and budgets of their units and related research programmes. Nurses, both as citizens and as professionals with special knowledge of the inside working of the National Health Service and of the practicalities of day-to-day health care, have a particular responsibility to speak out on issues of resource allocation.

The issues of resource allocation in health care refer not only to the expenditure of money on life-saving medical or surgical procedures and of high-technology equipment such as whole-body scanners or kidney dialysis machines, they refer also to expenditure on staff salaries, to the cost of building and equipping new hospitals or rebuilding and refurbishing old hospitals, to the cost of medical research, expenditure on drugs and disposable medical supplies and on such homely things as furniture, fittings and food. To put the 'expense' of controversial new medical procedures or life-saving medical intervention into perspective, it is necessary for nurses in general, and nurse managers in particular, to be well informed about the actual costs of the health services in their region, and nationally. In the next section some of the salient facts for health services in Scotland are outlined, in order to illustrate some of the areas of potential conflict in decision-making over resources in the National Health Service in Britain.

8.4 Vital statistics: their ethical and political implications

In exploring some 'political' responsibilities of the nurse, it may be helpful to examine some salient economic, demographic and epidemiological facts, and to consider the ethical implications for nursing services generally and for individual nurses in particular (Table 8.1).

Table 8.1 Vital statistics for Scotland and the United Kingdom for 1975 and 1985. (Compiled from ISD 1987, OPCS 1987, HMSO 1987)

	Scotland 1975	1985	United Kingdom 1975	1985
Total population	5.2 m	5.1 m	56.2 m	56.6 m = 100%
Males (M)	2.5 m	2.475 m	27.4 m	27.6
Females (F)	2.7 m	2.625 m	28.9 m	29.0
Under 5 years	7.2%	6.3%	6.6%	6.5%
0–15 years	26.3%	21.1%	24.9%	20.8%
16–64 years	60.5%	64.6%	61.1%	64.1%
65–74 years	8.7%	8.4%	9.0%	8.7%
75 years, and over	4.5%	5.9%	5.0%	6.4%
Live births/1000	13.1	13.0	12.4	13.3
Fertility rate	1.9	1.7	1.8	1.8
Deaths/1000 (M)	12.8	12.6	12.2	12.0
Deaths/1000 (F)	11.5	12.4	11.3	11.7
Percentages of all deaths:				
Heart disease	33.7%	34.4%	33.7%	33.0%
Cancers of all kinds	20.9%	22.9%	21.1%	23.8%
Motor vehicle accidents	1.3%	1.0%	1.0%	0.8%
Legal abortions	8,381	9,917	115,700	150,200
Life expectancy at birth (years)				
Males	67.8	70.0	69.9	71.8
Females	74.3	75.8	76.0	77.7

On the surface, the figures in Table 8.1 might not appear very interesting, but a closer look will reveal all sorts of hidden implications for future services and training.

First, note that the overall population of Scotland has been steadily declining over the past 10 years, whereas the UK population after a period of decline is beginning to increase again. On the one hand, this fall in population might be regarded as a triumph of sound family planning and good health education. In the other hand, it could signal a continuing fall in the future youthful population. Put in selfish terms, will there be enough economically active young people around to work and care for us when we reach retiring age? Either way, the figures have ethical and political implications for research and development, for the planning of services and for training.

The second major issue raised by the statistics set out in Table 8.1 relates to the growing proportion of people aged 75 years and over, the people who suffer the multiple pathologies of old age and who make heavy demands on the health and social services. The facts are that the largest proportion of hospital beds are occupied by patients over the age of 65 years, that there is an alarming increase in the number of elderly people needing psychiatric care, and that there is a vast increase in the numbers and proportion of the elderly in the community. Infant mortality rates have been dramatically reduced in this century and relatively few deaths occur in middle age, and today, for the first time in history, most dying is done by the elderly. Elderly people are more likely to die in hospital, so that death is increasingly unfamiliar (does not occur in the family).

The altered scene has already been recognised and reflected in health services planning and to some degree in a changed emphasis in training, but a great deal more needs to be done. While it may be an exaggeration to say that nurses and social workers enter these professions to work with children and end up working with elderly people, studies of student attitudes and expectations and the general bias of training confirms this, as well as the continuing high status accorded hi-tech and intensive care nursing above psychiatric and chronic care nursing (with the exception of terminal care nursing).

The statistics in Table 8.1 illustrating percentages of all deaths are, of course, vitally important for health education and the preventive services. Heart disease, respiratory diseases, and many forms of cancers are related to people's habits, lifestyles and to environmental factors — unlike the infectious diseases of the past. While the current AIDS epidemic has raised the spectre of past pandemics, the very nature of the disease and the circumstances of its transmission (mainly by sexual intercourse and intravenous drug abuse) indicates that its prevention is also crucially related to changing people's lifestyles. As already mentioned in Chapter 4, health education raises important questions about the rights and duties of the state and health professionals to intervene to change people's lifestyles. The political economy of health cannot be a matter of indifference to nurses.

When inappropriate diet, alcohol abuse and lack of exercise are implicated as causes of coronary heart disease and other diseases of the circulatory system, the pressure exerted on governments by the food and agriculture industries cannot be ignored. While we spend £16.5 billion on the National Health Service and are told that we cannot afford this level of public expenditure, we spend £15.8 billion per annum on alcohol and £7 billion on cigarettes and tobacco products. The Exchequer benefits to the tune of £5.2 billion from excise duty and tax on alcohol, but the estimated cost of alcohol abuse is £1.15 billion. The meagre resources for health education in Britain — an annual budget of under £20 million in 1985, compared with £650 million spent on advertising alcohol and tobacco. While Scots spend on average £3.4 million per day on alcohol and the total *annual* budget for health education is only £3.1 million, not a great deal can be done.

While legal abortions in 1985 accounted for only 0.19% of deaths in Scotland, the figure for the UK as a whole was 0.265%, and the total of 150 200 legal abortions in 1985 represented an increase of 30% over the figure for 1975. Whatever a person's moral convictions may be about the ethics of abortion, these figures are cause for concern — concern that so many unwanted pregnancies occur, that so many women have reason to terminate their pregnancies, that there are so many failures of contraception or failure to use any form of contraception. All these issues must be of concern to nurses, not only because they have to make choices about assisting or not assisting at terminations, but more fundamentally because midwives and health visitors are the frontline health educators in these matters. Again, there are many economic and political factors — relating to the status of women, the working conditions and terms of employment of women, and environmental and social factors — which complicate the whole problem. These factors must also be of concern to nurses, or they will be confined to providing 'sticking plaster' first aid in crisis response and crisis management instead of primary prevention of these painful human problems.

The costs of the National Health Service and related services (Table 8.2) is another area in which nurses would fail in their duty if they abrogated to others responsibility to share

Table 8.2 Costs of health services, 1975 and 1985

	Scotland 1975	Scotland 1985	United Kingdom 1985
Total cost	£591 m	£1963 m	£19 747 m
NI contributions	£45.5 m	£176.9 m	
Exchequer	£545.9 m	£1775.9 m	
Health board administration	£23.5 m	£55.5 m	£11 725 m
Hospital and community services:			
Revenue	£389.3 m	£1297 m	
Capital	£38.9 m	£117.8 m	
Hospital running costs	£358.0 m	£611.4 m	
Salaries:			
Medical and dental	£37.0 m	£127.5 m	
Nursing	£128.8 m	£436.0 m	
Community nursing	£35.9 m	£49.5 m	
Family practitioners	£101.3 m	£365.8 m	£4 277 m
Central health services:			
Revenue	£15.3 m	£53.3 m	
Capital	£3.6 m	£11.6 m	
Ambulance service	£7.8 m	£24.9 m	
Blood transfusion	£3.4 m	£13.4 m	
Health education	£0.5 m	£3.0 m	£15 m
Adminstration	£0.3 m	£2.1 m	
Training	£4.2 m	£15.3 m	
Research	£2.6 m	£5.3 m	

in public debate (and sometimes direct political activity) relating to health service policy, key problems affecting nursing services, and standards of patient care. Notable changes in the distribution of costs here are, first, the fact that 7.2% of the cost of the NHS in Scotland was paid for from National Insurance Contributions in 1975 compared with 9.2% in 1985, with proportional reduction in the contribution of the Exchequer. In the same period, costs of administration of health boards in Scotland were reduced from 5.5% to 3.9% of total costs. The proportion of total expenditure on nurses salaries increased from 21.8% to 22.2%. The proportion spent on health education did increase as well — from 0.08% to 0.15%, that is, from 9.6 p per head per annum to 58.8 p.

In Scotland, the Health Services Planning Council produced guidelines for the redistribution of manpower and resources during the 1980s, *Scottish Health Authorities Priorities for the Eighties* (SHHD 1980). In this report existing services were divided into three categories, A, B, C according to their priority, and indications were given of what the likely cost and staffing implications were of the changes proposed in shifting resources from other sectors.

— Category A: Prevention; Services for the multiply deprived; Care of the elderly; Elderly with mental disability; Mentally ill; Mental and physical handicap
— Category B: Maternity services; Primary dental care
— Category C: Child health; Acute hospital services.

Attempts have been made in recent Scottish health statistics to establish whether the SHAPE recommendations were being implemented, and to what extent (Table 8.3).

Table 8.3 Comparison of SHAPE categories 1980 and 1985

	1980	1985	% Change	1980	1985	% Change
	Hospital beds			Nursing staff		
Care of elderly	9 764	10 690	>9.5			
Psychogeriatric	2 742	3 765	>37.3			
Mental illness	17 040	16 307	<4.3	9 752	10 370	>6.3
Mental handicap	6 617	6 016	<9.1	3 428	3 711	>8.3
Physical handicap	470	536	>14.0			
Maternity	2 689	2 563	<4.7	4 593	4 673	>1.7
Maternal neonatal	3 315	3 142	<5.2	4 593	4 673	>1.7
Child health	1 257	1 173	<6.7			
General/acute	19 745	18 470	<6.5	35 479	37 986	>7.1
Total	58 208	56 334	<3.2	53 251	56 741	>6.6
Community nursing	4 907	5 238	>6.7			
Family practitioners	3 256	3 575	>9.8			
Dentists	1 280	1 407	>9.9			
Ophthalmic services	583	776	>33.1			
Pharmacists	1 107	1 134	>2.4			

The facts and figures alone do not enable us to decide on priorities in resource allocation. The duty to care and considerations of justice and the rights of patients are all relevant to the debate and the different weightings given to these principles influence policy about resource allocation in profound and subtle ways. Clearly, in making decisions about policy, and in attempting to influence policy at local and national level, different nurses will have different priorities, based on ethical principles and political leanings. However, they cannot responsibly avoid contributing to debate about these issues.

Doctors and nurses, trained to deal with the patients who present to them for care and treatment and trained in crisis management, naturally tend to see their first priority as being to save life. Their conditioned reflexes are to give priority to the duty to care — in a response which emphasises their sense of commitment to the individual patient — a clinical rather than an epidemiological view of the problem, and a personalist rather than an organisational set of values. Where the public is at risk in, say, an epidemic, or where medical research has to be undertaken in the interests of all patients, the duty to care for the individual has to be qualified by consideration of the rights of others and justice in the allocation of resources.

When Professor Chantler complains of the risks to children of inadequate resources for the treatment of victims of kidney disease, we see the tension illustrated in his emotive appeal for more resources for life-saving transplant surgery and dialysis machines, while he also admits the need for expenditure on prevention. In a sense he wants to have it both ways — unlimited resources to back up his strong sense of the duty to care for those whose lives are at risk, and further resources for prevention (in justice to the whole population who might become at risk but of whom those affected are only a tiny proportion). Dr Draper's case is based on epidemiological arguments, concerning changes in the pattern of mortality and morbidity in society. Here the control of infectious diseases and effective medical treatment of many life-threatening conditions has left the vast majority of people affected by disorders which are the chronic result of their lifestyle — respiratory disorders and lung cancer caused by smoking, diseases of the circulatory system caused by poor diet, lack of exercise, smoking and alcohol abuse, etc. The argument, based on considerations of justice in the interests of the majority, suggests that priority in the allocation of resources should be given to health education and prevention.

Even if the dilemma in dealing with coronary artery disease

and kidney disease could be resolved on the basis that because most cases of both diseases are preventable, priority should therefore be given to allocating resources to prevention rather than treatment, this still leaves the dilemmas related to the treatment of defective newborns or the rights of childless couples unanswered.

While it is possible by antenatal diagnosis to determine whether a fetus is defective, and so to offer the parents the possibility of abortion as an alternative to bearing a child with Down's syndrome or spina bifida, there are nevertheless (despite questions which may be raised about abortion) still many cases where antenatal tests have not been done or the test refused. Here, faced with a case of a spina bifida baby with even a limited hope of survival, the right of the child to treatment and the duty to care by the doctor and nursing staff would seem to override any abstract considerations of justice for others, when faced with the concrete case of a child needing emergency treatment and care.

The right of infertile couples to medical assistance in seeking to have a child would seem to many people to be fundamental. However, the paradox is that the helpless defective newborn whose *prima facie* right to treatment may seem so obvious and to whom the staff may be thought to owe a primary duty to care, may be denied life-saving treatment because it is thought to be unjust to burden a family (or society) with a severely handicapped individual who will make great demands on social resources. In contrast to the helpless infant who is unable to argue his case, forceful articulate and determined couples may be able to exert great pressure on medical and nursing staff to recognise their rights and meet their demands. In both cases, difficult decisions may have to be made and these relate to setting limits to what it is reasonable and just for the public to demand of the health services, medical and nursing staff, in view of other demands on time, manpower and financial resources.

The objective assessment of the malformed baby's prospects for survival and quality of life have to be balanced against what burden of responsibility it is reasonable and practicable to expect the medical and nursing staff, the child's parents and society to carry. Justice demands that these other interests should be taken into account in deciding whether expensive life-saving measures should be taken.

In the case of the childless couple there may well have to be limits set to what it is fair to expect public health services to provide. Given the low level of risk involved in remaining childless, it might be argued that, in spite of the emotional cost to the young couple, and the possible risk to their marriage, their 'right' to have a child should not be given priority over other more préssing needs of patients with life-threatening conditions or where saving the life of premature babies is concerned. Treatment for infertility may even be regarded as a luxury when the aim is to limit fertility in the interests of population control and the conservation of diminishing global resources; and in the Third World countries the attempt to set up such services would hardly even be considered. However, it could also be argued that since the knowledge and technology exists to assist many childless couples to have children, whether by *in vitro* fertilisation or by some other means such as surrogate parenthood, in a prosperous society, like Britain, this help should be available through the National Health Service; alternatively, people should be able to get the help privately if they can afford it or can raise the money from charity. Even then would it be reasonable to expect medical and nursing staff to give up time and resources to meet further demands, for example that a couple be provided specifically with a daughter with particular genetic endowment, such as beauty, intelligence and musical ability? Or that they be assisted to choose an indefinite number of copies of themselves?

Discussion of these examples illustrates how in such cases it is necessary to strike a balance between the demands of beneficence, respect for persons and justice.

8.5 The nurse as an agent of health and social policy

In discussing the ethics of resource allocation in health care, Boyd (1979) examined four different approaches to decision-making in this area, which he identified as: Ecological and Epidemiological; Clinical; Administrative; and Egalitarian. However, these four approaches may be interpreted more broadly as applying to other areas of decision-making in health care, relating to wider social and political issues as well. In discussing the nurse as an agent of health and social policy it will be useful to bear these categories in mind. We will consider the attitude of nurses and their duty to contribute in a responsible way to public debate about the question of how the Health Service is to be funded, the issue of private medicine either within or as an alternative to the National Health Service, the priority to be given to health education, the relative importance of high-technology medicine and advanced research in exotic areas of medicine, and the need for better primary medical care and community services.

Clinical approach. In the previous section it was argued that doctors and nurses are not primarily trained as administrators, and that they tend to understand their responsibilities primarily in terms of the duty to care rather than in terms of the rights of patients and health care for the whole society. This approach emphasises the special knowledge and expertise of health professionals and their presumed right to special authority in decision-making about matters related to health care. The limitations of such an approach are that it tends to be individualistic in dealing with problems which may have complex social origins and consequences; it tends to be crisis-oriented, with emphasis on the importance of curative medicine and medical research rather than prevention; it tends to be clinically and morally authoritarian, underplaying the expertise of other professionals and presuming that special moral insight is available to clinicians yet denied to others.

Epidemiological approach. Based on a study of the changing pattern of mortality and morbidity in society, the epidemiological approach is more concerned to emphasise the need for objective consideration of health priorities in the light of demonstrable trends in the relative incidence and prevalence of different disorders. The emphasis on these more objective and universal considerations tends to be based on a concept of a rational justice for all, rather than on respect for the rights of individuals or the duty to care. Given the evidence marshalled by individuals such as McKeown (1976), that the decrease in infant mortality and the control of infectious diseases was brought about more by sanitary measures, public health legislation and improvements in diet and housing than by direct medical intervention, it is argued that less priority should be given to the acute medical services and more to community medicine and health education. Furthermore, the fact that most mortality and morbidity in contemporary developed countries is lifestyle-related, strengthens the argument for primacy to be given to prevention of disease (HMSO 1976, SHHD 1980). However, the power of entrenched medical interests is shown in the fact that cuts are being made at the expense of preventive medicine and the caring services.

The limitations of the epidemiological approach are that it is too abstract and impersonal, too far removed from the emotive reality of individual suffering and the demands of individuals to have their rights respected. It underestimates the effect of 'miraculous' cures on the public imagination and the limited impact or credibility of the invisible influence of prevention. It also tends to be too far removed from such social realities as poverty, deprivation and ignorance which provide the background to ill-health in contemporary society, and it tends to underestimate the countervailing irrational forces which strengthen patterns of unhealthy living, including stress and anxiety, economic insecurity and the influence of advertisements.

Administrative approach. The model which preoccupies those who adopt this approach is that of the health services as an industry, as a service industry with a specific contract to provide health services to health-service consumers in return for payment based on fees, taxation or health insurance. The assumptions are that in the market for services the client can negotiate his treatment with the health professionals and that health provision can be rationally planned on the basis of supply and demand. The effectiveness of medical procedures will, according to this model, be based on proper scientific tests, randomised trials and controlled experimentation. The tests of efficiency will be the relative costs and benefits of alternative procedures, measured in terms of productivity like any other industry — for example, by bed turnover or discharge rates. The administrative model gives particular emphasis to organisational and scientific rationality and to the contractual rights of patients and the duties of health professionals based on a business model.

In many respects this approach is a refreshing change from the beneficent paternalism of the clinical model and the implicitly authoritarian paternalism of the epidemiological model. It emphasises the autonomy of the patient and the objectivity of his rights, but it tends to ignore the fact that the provision of medical and nursing care is not just a commercial transaction like that with any other service industry. The relationship between the contracting parties is inherently unequal and the vulnerability and dependence of the patient demands a quality of trustworthy responsibility on the part of the health professional which is unique, because people's lives and health are at stake.

Egalitarian approach. In line with a more political and radical approach to social justice in health care, the emphasis here is on the necessity for changes in the socio-economic structure of society. Active policies of community development and positive discrimination in favour of the socially deprived are imperative, if inequalities in health are to be overcome.

The Black Report (DHSS 1980) illustrates, with a wealth of facts and statistics, two basic theses: first, that the nationalisation of the Health Service brought great benefits to British society in the dramatic improvement of the average level of health of the population and in the more equal distribution of health care and resources; second, that between the extremes, in social class terms, the gap has widened in terms of a whole range of health indicators from infant mortality to indices for common causes of mortality that are lifestyle-related. The apparent contradiction between these two theses is explained by the fact that the greater proportion of the population is now in social classes III and IV and less in social class V than in 1947. The general tenor of the report is accordingly that the NHS has been a good thing, but that it needs to be improved and that greater resources should be put into areas of serious social deprivation if a real impact is to be made in improving the disparities in health between social classes I and V.

The Black Report was damned with faint praise by Patrick

Jenkin, then Minister of Health in the Conservative Government, and most of its recommendations have been ignored,
although comparable evidence has not been marshalled in
support of the alternative policies. If the tendency to blame
the victim is to be answered, then it has to be met by a
number of strategies. Appeal to facts and evidence is one.
Emphasis on the duty to care and the respect due to the rights
of the poor is another. Appeals to justice are not enough, if
they are not motivated by beneficence and respect for
persons.

Nurses following a narrow clinical model may favour private
medicine because the quality of care for the few patients in
such units may be much better than in the NHS. But the nurse
cannot, as a responsible health professional, be solely
concerned about 'her' patients and her income. She must
surely, in justice and respect for the rights of all patients, be
concerned about the ones who cannot afford private medicine and suffer discrimination because the better-off can
afford to 'jump the queue'. However, if she sincerely believes
that the interests of justice and respect for the rights of all
patients are better served by private medicine then she has an
obligation to produce the evidence and reasons in support of
her view. In the absence of such reasons and evidence, that
of the Royal Commission on the National Health Service and
the evidence of great disparities in the standards of health
care for rich and poor in countries like the USA may convince
her, against the alleged primacy of her duty to care for 'her'
patients or the alleged 'rights' of the rich to buy a better standard of care. If it can be demonstrated that the rich can enjoy
that right without associated prejudice to the standard of care
enjoyed by others, and that has yet to be demonstrated, then
that might be a practical alternative (Campbell 1978).

In discussing each of the questions posed — regarding
funding of the National Health Service, preventive or curative
medicine, the relative importance of high technology, acute
medicine and advanced medical research versus the provision
of better primary and community care — perhaps none of the
four models taken by itself is adequate. Discussed against the
background of three complementary moral principles each
model has to be qualified. Politics, as Aristotle observed, is
the art of the possible; or, as he suggested in another

context, it is the attempt to find the best means to achieve good ends in the light both of our principles and practical experience. This means that the pleasure of politics lies in the creativity of finding new and and better solutions to old problems, but the burden is also that of knowing that no solution will be ideal and that our principles may have to be compromised to some degree because of the intractibility of reality and human nature.

REFERENCES

Boyd K M 1979 The ethics of resource allocation in health care. Edinburgh University Press, Edinburgh
Campbell A V 1978 Medicine, health and justice: The problem of priorities. Churchill Livingstone, Edinburgh
DHSS 1980 Inequalities in health: Report of a commission of enquiry into the National Health Service (Chairman: Sir Douglas Black). Department of Health and Social Security, London
Draper P, Popay J 1980 Medical charities, prevention and the media. British Medical Journal 280, 110
Dworkin G 1977 Strikes and the National Health Service. Journal of Medical Ethics 3(2), 75–85
Eadie H A (1975): 'The Helping Personality': CONTACT, Number 49, Summer.
Feifel H et al 1967 Physicians consider death. Proceedings of American Psychological Association conv. 201–2
Freidson E 1970 Profession of Medicine. Dodd Mead, New York
HMSO 1976 Prevention and health — everybody's business. Her Majesty's Stationery Office, London
HMSO 1978 Report of the enquiry into Normansfield Hospital, Cmnd 7357. Her Majesty's Stationery Office, London
HMSO 1987 Social trends 17. Her Majesty's Stationery Office, London
ISD 1987 Scottish health statistics. Advance tables 1987. Common Services Agency, Edinburgh
McKeown T 1976 The role of medicine. Nuffield Provincial Hospitals Trust, London
OPCS 1987 Monitor, reference DH2 87/3, 8 Sept. Office of Population Censuses and Surveys, London
RCN 1977 Code of Professional Conduct: A discussion document. Journal of Medical Ethics 3(3), 121
SHHD 1980 Scottish health authorities' priorities for the eighties. HMSO, Edinburgh

9

Moral decision-making

9.1 Taking moral decisions

It was remarked in Chapter 5 that, when thinking about ethics, we tend to focus on the big dilemmas, the urgent and dangerous situations where we have to take big and risky decisions. While it is understandable that attention should focus on painful problems and the difficulty experienced in taking decisions relating to them, it does tend to skew our perception of decision-making, for in everyday life and in routine work we take decisions with little awareness of doing so. It is interesting that in Greek the word 'crisis' originally just meant 'decision-time', a time when we have to make a judgement about what to do next. Obviously, when we are faced with life-threatening and urgent problems and have to do something, we are faced with a crisis — the urgent need to take a decision. The word crisis refers also to major turning points in our lives — or in the course of an illness — and often it is because these events are also associated with making painful decisions. However, most decisions we take are neither dramatic nor dangerous. In performing routine work numerous minor decisions are taken every day, including numerous routine moral decisions.

It is important to stress that not all moral decision-making is associated with drama and crisis. On the contrary, most of

us develop remarkable skill at making rapid moral assessments of the practical situations in our life and in taking the
appropriate decisions. Some decision times will be crises for
us, but like the advertising slogan it is important generally
'not to make a drama out of a crisis'.

In general, our ordinary upbringing in family, school, work
and the wider community equips us with knowledge of the
moral values and rules in our society and with practical skills
to apply them. Some of these values and rules we will adopt
as our own, others we may simply respect to the extent that
is necessary to get on with people, but others again we may
actively criticise or reject. Whatever we do and whichever lifestyle we choose, our decisions and actions, our moral judgements, will embody and express our *value judgements*. Like
learning to walk or run, where we employ the principles of
physiology, mechanics and kinaesthetics without being aware
of these, in routine decision-making we are applying scientific, organisational and moral principles in a highly complex
process which we would find as difficult to explain as the man
challenged to explain how he manages to walk (Toulmin 1958,
Campbell & Higgs 1982).

We do not normally reflect critically on what we are doing
when we make decisions, particularly those decisions which
embody and express established moral values, unless faced
with a crisis. In this sense a 'crisis' may be interpreted as a
situation which *demands a decision*, but where the nature of
the circumstances also challenges or forces us to reflect on
what we are doing and perhaps even to give a clear explanation of our reasons for deciding and acting as we do.

Several factors may cause us to experience decision-time as
a crisis. The first is where we are entering unfamiliar territory
— for example, when the trainee nurse first encounters the
practical and moral problems of nursing, or when the experienced nurse acquires new responsiblity. Here, lack of appropriate knowledge or skills, unfamiliarity with established rules
of practice or ignorance of likely outcomes may undermine
the confidence of nurses and force them to examine carefully
what they are doing and why. Related to this is a second kind
of crisis, namely where an individual suddenly finds himself
faced with greater-than-usual responsibility, or is obliged to
act on his own without the usual opportunities to check

things out with colleagues or friends. Here the urgency of the problem that has to be dealt with and the need to accept responsibility oneself may challenge one to seek a clear justification for what one has done so as to be able to answer criticism if things go wrong. The third point concerns the nature of decision itself — namely, that choosing one thing or one course of action forecloses other options. (The word 'decision', coming from the same root as 'incision', has the connotation of cutting off other possibilities.) Deciding to accept one job rather than another or to marry one person rather than another has long-term implications for one's life and limits other decisions. Faced with situations where decisions are irreversible or where the consequences will be far-reaching, we may also be forced to pause and reflect. A fourth situation is the genuine moral dilemma — a conflict of duties or a painful choice between two equally unacceptable moral outcomes. Here we are forced to reflect critically, not on the circumstances in which the decision is demanded, nor on the degree of responsibility demanded of us, nor on the likely consequences, but on our moral principles as such, how they are related and which are to have priority, if that determination is possible.

Another kind of challenge which can force us to re-examine our whole moral position is when someone demands that we justify our fundamental moral principles and values, or when some event in our lives causes us to call in to question and to doubt the whole basis of our moral beliefs. We are forced back to a more basic level where we are obliged to examine the presuppositions on which our moral beliefs are based and the reasons and evidence we could produce to justify them. While confrontation by another person or a personal crisis may be painful challenges to our moral theory, the discipline of philosophy is a systematic way in which we can study these questions and test solutions against those worked out by others over the centuries. This particular aspect of decision-making — namely, that concerned with moral theory and the justification of our fundamental moral principles — is the subject of the final chapter of this book. At this stage, however, we return to the analysis and description of the more basic characteristics of routine decision-making.

9.2 Conscience, feeling, intuition and moral judgement

Since we do, in fact, make moral judgements all the time — about what we consider right and wrong in general, what we consider the best course of action in a specific situation — or make judgements about our own or other people's actions and characters (and we do this semi-automatically), we tend to resist attempts to analyse the process involved. We appeal to 'the voice of conscience' or 'intuition', or say that 'it just felt right'.

In the first place, these phrases refer to a genuine sense that in our experience moral judgement, decision and action are as natural a part of living and doing as breathing. Because our moral experience is co-extensive with the rest of our human experience and permeates all we are and do, it is perhaps a rather artificial exercise to try and separate it out. We adopt values, making them our own. We learn habitual responses and forms of action, so that they become 'second nature' to us. Virtue and vice are habitual dispositions of thought and action, like the skilled and graceful performance of the trained gymnast on the one hand or the self-destructive lifestyle of someone who habitually depends on drugs or alcohol on the other (Thomson 1976).

Appeal to conscience or intuition can also be a form of mystification — suggesting that decision-making is a kind of impalpable and private, even occult, process. The discussion at this point often echoes the school of thought which claims that 'nurses are born not made', that the attributes of nursing — empathy and sympathy, sensitivity to the patient's real needs, gentleness, competence, efficiency — cannot be taught. Of course, some people have natural predispositions to care, and others have not, but if we can rationally understand and describe what these skills consist of, then in principle they can also be taught. Likewise, some people may start with certain advantages of moral upbringing, experience and practical wisdom and may therefore appear more competent and confident in making decisions and exercising moral responsibility. While even the most confident person can be shaken in a crisis, it is equally true that most people can be trained to carry responsibility and learn to cope with routine crises.

In ethics, it is important to demystify moral decision-making, both for the sake of clarity and truth and to encourage people to address those forms of knowledge and skill which can be learned and taught. Moral decision-making is just another form of problem-solving activity, and the models we apply to other forms of problem-solving are equally relevant here. The Nursing Process, besides being a method of planning nursing care in an intelligent and rational way, represents a way of demystifying nursing care. Rigid and unimaginative following through of the Nursing Process will not guarantee either the quality of care or the competence with which it is given. The method presupposes the application of knowledge and intelligence, skill and sensitivity to the needs of the patient in the particular situation. The knowledge and skills can perhaps be directly taught, but the commonsense and sensitivity are not so much 'taught' as 'caught' — by imitation of others with more experience of life and practical wisdom. Similarly, the application of decision-making models or theory to moral judgement does not guarantee that the decision taken will be either wise or morally sound. Following a method, analysing a decision or planning a course of action in a systematic way only ensures that it is done in a more rational manner and enables clearer reasons and coherent justification to be given for what has been done. Acting responsibly means being able to give an account of what has been done, that is, accepting that you are liable to have to give sound reasons for your actions. Following an appropriate problem-solving method for making moral decisions will considerably help in demonstrating intelligent and practical accountability (Campbell & Higgs 1982, Downie & Calman 1987).

It is perhaps worth pausing to consider the origin of expressions like 'conscience', 'intuition' and 'feeling'. While the 'voice of conscience' may mean anything from the echo of parental authority to Freud's super-ego or the voice of God, the inner voice of conscience seems to refer, on the one hand, to the sense of conviction we have about our moral beliefs and the authority they have for us in deciding what is right and wrong. On the other hand, 'conscience' seems to stand for collected and collective moral wisdom or practical experience which lends weight to our feeling that a course of action is right. However, it is noteworthy that the original meaning of the word 'conscience' (from Latin *cum*, with, and *scientia*, knowledge) means 'having comprehensive theoretical and practical knowledge'. Conscience in the classical sense is that faculty which integrates awareness of moral values with theoretical knowledge and practical experience, enabling a circumspect view of things before action. The same could be said of the word 'intuition', which has been interpreted as an integrative ability of the imagination to take the confusing variety of data and phenomena in a situation and make some kind of sense out of them. The faculty of intuition not only helps us to locate our experience in space and time, in relation to preceding and subsequent events and other similar or different situations, but also carries the suggestion that enables us to imagine the possible outcomes of alternative courses of action. 'Feeling things are right' is not necessarily or exclusively a statement about private feelings, but can also be taken to refer to the sense of 'having one's bearings' of being oriented, having a sense of direction about where one is going — a settled conviction that in relation to what you know and your past experience this is the most appropriate thing to do (Campbell 1984).

Exploring what is meant by decision-making in terms of 'conscience', 'intuition' and 'feeling' can only lead so far. But if we consider the model of the Nursing Process or other models for problem-solving, we can perhaps see more specifically what is involved in moral decision-making. The stages can be set out as follows: Assessment of the problem situation; Planning what to do about it; Implementing the planned decision; Evaluating the success of your action (Roper et al 1981).

9.3 Practical models for moral decision-making: Analogy with the Nursing Process

In the context of nursing care the application of the Nursing Process is not simply a technical method of directing clinical practice in terms of rational care plans, as if moral considerations did not come into it. In any care plan or application of the Nursing Process all sorts of moral considerations are both taken for granted and often explicit. The purpose of pursuing this analogy with the Nursing Process in analysing moral decision-making is not only practical, in seeking to clarify the processes involved, it is also to stress that the nurse's moral experience and nursing experience are one and the same. But what, then, are the practical implications of the applications of this model to the analysis of the moral aspects of decision-making in nursing?

Assessment

Just as the nurse is expected to take a detailed history from patients and carefully note their general circumstances as well as the specific problems they are experiencing, and to apply her general knowledge of the principles and practice of nursing to the interpretation and assessment of the situation, so a similar process is involved in making moral decisions.

First, we have to clarify what conditions prevail in the different circumstances; for example, a community nurse visiting a bedbound elderly patient at home, or a casualty nurse in an ambulance team attending victims of a railway accident in a remote place, or a nursing officer dealing with acutely ill patients in an understaffed ward. In the first case, it may be as important for the district nurse to have good knowledge of the housing conditions, financial state and family supports (or lack of them) of the bedbound patient as it would be to know what resources could be called upon to assist in providing good nursing care. What effective care can be given, and even what it would be right or wrong to do, in emergency first aid to accident victims in a remote place, where only minimal medical resources are available, will be determined and limited by the circumstances. The problems of the nursing officer faced with staffing shortages and the duty to care for acutely ill patients are only clarified by careful analysis of what the real needs of patients are, what resources are available and what is actually possible.

Secondly, we have to clarify what kind of knowledge and skills are relevant in deciding what to do. This will include relevant rules and moral principles relating to one's personal and professional duties. Merely to provide nursing care for the bedbound patient (for example, to administer a routine bedbath or pain relief, or to recommend hospitalisation) would be irresponsible if no attempt was made to ensure that family members provided what support they could manage. The same would apply if the patient's right to a home-help, disability allowance and provision of physical aids was not respected. The principle of beneficence, or the duty to care, interpreted narrowly, would not be sufficient to clarify what should be done. In the case of the railway accident, where those giving assistance would possibly have to apply a policy of triage (leaving those who are too far gone for help and those who are likely to recover without help, and concentrating efforts on those who have a chance of recovery but are unlikely to do so without help), the demands of the duty to care may have to take precedence over considerations of justice or respect for the rights of individuals. A nursing officer without sufficient staff to operate an acute ward, by contrast, might have to take political action — for example, threatening to walk out unless help is urgently forthcoming. Here a nurse's action might be guided by considerations of justice and respect for the right of all committed into her care.

Planning

Once the problem has been clearly defined (by a careful assessment of the general circumstances, the needs of the specific individual/s, and the general nursing and moral principles relevant to the situation), then it may be possible to plan a course of action. This will involve several stages:

— Consideration of the specific knowledge and practical procedures known be relevant to the defined problem
— Retrospective examination of past experience of the success or failure of alternative courses of action for dealing with similar problems
— Prospective anticipation of the likely consequences of alternative courses of action in this specific situation
— Choice of appropriate means to achieve the desired goal, including ensuring that appropriate resources are available
— Formulating a plan of action, including possible contingency plans if things go wrong and circumstances allow a change of plan.

Ability to make sound action plans requires the particular combination of knowledge, skill and practical experience that we call practical wisdom or what Aristotle and the classical philosophers called the virtue of prudence — namely the ability to choose the right *means* (in the light of moral *principles* to achieve a good *end* (outcome or goal) (Thomson 1976). However, having a good plan and all the experience of a lifetime cannot protect against the unexpected or chance developments that may throw everything awry. Prudence requires flexibility and adaptability too, and good planning will allow for contingencies as well (Pieper 1959).

Implementation

How effectively and efficiently decisions are implemented, and plans worked out in practice will have a great deal to do with their success or failure. Aristotle identified a specific virtue or skill (*solertia*) which is associated with being confident, decisive and courageous in carrying through a decision or action plan. This virtue is something certain people learn with experience, enabling them to avoid timorousness and indecisiveness, while nevertheless remaining sensitively responsive to changing situations without being overrigid in keeping to their plans at all costs (Pieper 1959).

Implementation is the key part of 'action', but it cannot be considered in isolation. From a moral point of view we are concerned with the soundness of the whole process. This includes responsible assessment of the general circumstances and principles relevant to a specific situation, the development of an appropriate action plan, the effective and efficient implementation of practical decisions, and the evaluation of the consequences or outcome in terms of specific goals, and general costs and benefits. At each stage, moral deliberation and judgement will involve consideration of relevant facts or knowledge, skills and values in terms of which we interpret and evaluate the appropriateness and sensitivity with which assessments are made.

Evaluation

The term 'evaluation' can be applied to the attempt to judge each stage in the process of decision-making, but it is more commonly used in a restricted sense to apply to consequences or outcomes. Evaluating a decision does certainly, and importantly, involve consideration of whether the actual consequences of an implemented plan of action are the same as the intended consequences, whether those consequences are better or worse than hoped for, and whether the long-term effects of a course of action would justify its becoming standard practice. Evaluation in this sense is part of a learning process. The feedback from experience, if consciously integrated into an understanding of what we are doing, should equip us to act better and more efficiently when faced with similar situations in the future. In this way the feedback in the learning process helps to build in habits which make decision making potentially easier as we gain in experience and confidence. However, there is a broader aspect of evaluation of importance to moral judgement. This relates to the cost/benefit analysis of alternative courses of action, not merely whether they are efficient in achieving our desired ends. Evaluation of costs and benefits is not simply a requirement of sound economics and practical management of professional tasks, it is also a demand of moral judgement. This brings us back full circle to the re-examination of the fundamental principles and values espoused in the belief that they promote human flourishing. In nursing, health promotion and promotion of 'complete physical, mental and social well-being' are one and the same activity. Moral considerations are inseparable from the Nursing Process!

Finally, there is the inclusive sense of evaluation. This covers the whole process of decision-making (including assessment, planning, implementation and evaluation). Evaluation is concerned both with judgements about how well individual steps in the process have been completed and how successfully the whole process has been in practical and moral terms. Ethical disagreements can arise at each of these stages in the process. There can be disputes about facts and values in relation to assessment of what ought to be done, how it should be done, how well it is actually done, and whether the specific outcomes or general consequences are good. The words 'ought', 'should', 'well', 'good' belong to the vocabulary of moral judgement and relate to rules, duties, and values for the assessment of performance and general costs and benefits respectively. As will be seen in the next chapter disputes at the level of moral theory relate to the different ways we justify our moral judgements in each of these contexts (Hare 1952, Nowell Smith 1957).

9.4 Practical models for decision-making: A sociological model

Four interrelated factors are involved in practical decision-making: the demands of the situation, the roles of the different participants, the variety of rules applicable, and the arbiters — or, more simply, situation, roles and rules, and arbiters. All these factors have to be taken into account. (Emmet 1966, Downie 1971).

Situation. The details of a moral situation are important. It will involve some general factors common to most human situations and some which are unique to this particular situation. In institutions such as hospitals there are general factors common to most patients: their vulnerability and dependency, their need for nursing care and medical treatment, their relative lack of privacy, and in a particular ward maybe the same kinds of medical problems. However, each individual has a unique medical history, specific identity and social status, a particular set of family or social obligations. Both general and specific factors in the situation, including those relating to the staff and available resources, need to be taken into account.

Roles and rules. These tend to be interconnected. The roles of patient, doctor, nurse, porter, administrator, relative, all tend to be governed by different specific and traditional rules of permissible and non-permissible behaviour, as well as general rules governing the institution, more general rules and laws governing society, and universal moral principles in terms of which we attempt to order and make sense of all these other rules. People in a given situation may play more than one role at a time. A patient, besides, being a patient, may be a father, a lawyer, a champion bridge-player and a protestant. The nurse may be a man, a qualified SNO, union member and Roman Catholic. The doctor may be a young woman, feminist, keen golfer and atheist. All these factors relating to roles and rules would be relevant in decision-making but to different degrees, depending on what was at issue (Downie 1971).

Arbiters. When we make moral decisions we also have to consider to whom we are responsible and accountable — in other words, the arbiters of our actions. The nurse would be responsible to the patient and responsible for the patient, to some extent (though not responsible for the patient in the same way as the doctor). Nurses are also accountable to their peers and superiors, to the doctor, and ultimately to the relatives and society. We invariably 'look over our shoulder' to consider who is watching our actions. Those people to whom we are collectively responsible and accountable, the arbiters of our actions, also have to be taken into account when we decide what to do.

Because all these factors are variable each situation is different, people play different roles, numerous different rules apply, and we are accountable to a variety of people in different ways. Moral decision-making is complex — especially in an institutional setting. Having the ability and confidence to make responsible decisions is a matter of knowledge, and growth in experience and sophistication, sensitivity and wisdom (Emmet 1966, Thompson 1979).

9.5 The moral agent: When is a person responsible for their actions?

In the fifth century BC Aristole pointed out that we do not apportion praise or blame for actions unless the person has acted knowingly and voluntarily. People cannot be held responsible for their actions if they acted involuntarily or in complete ignorance of what they were doing or what the consequences of their actions were likely to be. Although we may want to refine his criteria, the commonsense rules suggested by Aristotle are still useful for most practical purposes (Thomson 1976).

Aristotle distinguished between voluntary, involuntary and non-voluntary actions. Voluntary acts are those knowingly and purposefully undertaken to achieve a particular goal — for example, forming and executing a plan to go to town to buy some clothes. Involuntary, or reflex, 'actions', such as jumping up with a shout of pain having sat on a sharp tack, or knocking a cup off the table because you withdraw your hand suddenly on contact with a hot kettle, are mechanical reactions, or forms of behaviour, resulting from internal or external causes which are neither purposeful nor subject to conscious control. Non-voluntary actions are actions which are done either in ignorance or a state of intoxication, when you are not fully aware of what you are doing or are compelled to do something against your will, — for example, at gunpoint or when subjected to forces you cannot control (Aristotle's example was of the ship's master who is forced to jettison his cargo in a storm to avoid his ship being swamped).

In general terms, we cannot be held fully responsible for actions which we did not cause but which we were caused to do by external factors or forces beyond our control. Determining the degree to which someone can be held responsible for their actions in a particular case will therefore involve careful assessment of the full circumstances in order to establish: whether the person acted knowingly or in ignorance; whether the person acted vountarily or not; whether the person was subject to external (or internal) compulsion.

When the person actively causes things to happen which would not have happened without their intervention, then we regard the person as the responsible agent. When a person is the passive object of external forces acting upon them, or simply reacts in a mechanical or reflexive way to external causes, then we do not regard the person as responsible. Obviously there may be difficulty in determining for certain the degree to which a given person acted freely or under duress in a particular situation, or to what extent their ignorance, state of intoxication or inner sense of compulsion could serve as excusing conditions if they were being tried for a serious crime. Making these assessments is part of the day-to-day business of juries and law courts, but also of the assessments of staff performance for disciplinary or promotion purposes. (Aristotle showed some interesting reservations in the treating of ignorance, drunkenness or inner compulsions as excusing conditions — regarding human beings as at least partially responsible for their own ignorance, excessive drinking or tendency to give way to irrational compulsion) (Downie 1971.)

The difficulty in assessing the degree to which 'voluntary' acts are actually 'free' acts — given the many factors which limit freedom and predetermine scope for action — may lead us to question more radically whether human beings are free at all. Do human beings have free will or are they wholly determined?

Before discussing the free-will/determinism controversy in outline it is important to note that both law and social morality rest on the assumption that people are normally responsible for their actions. Those wishing to plead diminished responsibility have to produce strong evidence that they were temporarily insane, incapacitated, acting under duress or the like. Excusing conditions in law or morality are offered by way of extenuating circumstances to lessen the degree of guilt or blame for an act, or to reduce the penalties exacted. Moral and legal discourse take for granted that it is possible to discriminate between voluntary and non-voluntary acts and reflex behaviour.

9.6 Free will and determinism — a philosophical 'red herring'?

Several ways lead to the view that while people may think they are free they are in reality wholly determined in what they do. We may believe that human beings are created and controlled by some superior being, or God, who wholly predetermines how we will act. We may believe that a universal law of causality operates in nature or the material world so that cause and effect are necessarily connected in such a way that effects follow inevitably and without exception from their causes. Or we may believe that we are programmed by our genetic constitution and the accidental circumstances of birth and upbringing so that everything we do is predictable.

The language of law and morality, as well as ordinary language itself, assumes the distinctions between active and passive moods, assumes that human beings can be both active agents initiating actions, or passive patients at the receiving end of the actions of others. For most ordinary purposes we describe our actions from the standpoint of actors or agents who do things for *reasons*, with definite aims or objectives in mind. When we explain our actions, stand back and reflect on how and why we acted as we did, we analyse the rules and evidence on which we operate. We may indicate external forces that caused us to act in a particular way, or we may seek to justify or excuse ourselves by pointing to particular features of our inherited constitution, experience (or ignorance), or limiting factors in our environment that restricted our freedom of choice. In attempting a retrospective analysis of past actions we adopt the standpoint of spectators towards our own actions. We see our actions as caused (or determined) by the complex reasons, facts, and evidence offered by way of explanation or justification of what we have done. When we attempt the same kind of analysis of the actions of other people, we are easily persuaded that the explanations of how and why they acted as they did are compelling; that, given foreknowledge of the person, their background and acquired knowledge and attitudes, and the prevailing circumstances, we could actually predict how they would behave. Husbands and wives, lovers and enemies often believe they know one another so well that they can predict exactly what the other will say or do. Strangely, if this were inevitably the case we would doubt that the other was really alive and not a robot.

From the fact that people have reasons for acting as they do, it does not follow that their reasons are the direct causes for things happening the way they do. Reasons are not to be confused with causes. Antecedent and consequent explanations of actions tend to have a different logic. The person who offers reasons for their acting in a particular way sees the events in terms of the self-determining action of himself/herself as a free agent. Retrospective analysis of causes, or of necessary and sufficient conditions for an action to occur, tends to define the events as determined, the outcome predictable, and the scope of choice limited. Rather like looking at the world through Alice's looking glass, determinist arguments see everything retrospectively through the frame of the spectator's mirror.

The type of theology which argues from the existence of an omnipotent, omniscient God to the conclusion that man cannot in any sense be free or responsible for his actions, because all his actions must be foreknown and therefore predestined by God, adopts the radical spectator point-of-view. The person who professes such a theological determinism assumes that they can personally adopt the privileged position of viewing man and the universe 'sub specie aeternitatis', from a God's-eye point-of-view, and declares that moral effort is pointless because everything is predetermined anyway. The argument assumes:

— If you have complete knowledge of someone (omniscience)
— If you can be constantly present to them (omnipresent)
— If you can comprehend and control all the variables in their lives and circumstances (omnipotence)
— Then you could determine in advance everything they would do.

The argument rests on a number of big 'ifs', but it also makes a dubious logical assumption, namely that foreknowledge is coercive or compelling of future outcomes.

The arguments for determinism which rest on the so-called Law of Universal Causation are particularly appealing to those who attempt to offer comprehensive scientific or historical explanations of world events, natural processes and the behaviour of human beings. These arguments rest on the faith that the Law of Universal Causation applies without exception throughout the universe. By its very nature this is an unverifiable metaphysical belief. It is tempting to extrapolate from causal processes in contained and finite systems to the universe as a whole; but this is not logically justified. Causal inference is a method we apply to the analysis of processes in nature that display predictable regularity. It is a conceptual tool which we freely apply to the ordering of our experience in an attempt to make sense of the world. We cannot argue that the choice to employ cause and effect explanations is itself determined by the law of cause and effect without getting into a circular argument.

The types of arguments developed in some forms of determinist psychology (e.g. Freudian or Behaviourist) or some forms of sociology (e.g. Marxist/Leninist) appear to offer very powerful explanations of why people behave in certain ways. For the Freudian, neurotic behaviour in adult life is directly caused by traumatic emotional disturbances in childhood, or, more generally, that human beings are inevitably determined by their particular heredity and environment. For the strict Behaviourist like Pavlov, all human and social action is the result of historical and economic forces acting upon individuals, over which they have no control. (That is, unless they have privileged access to the higher truth and insights of dialectical materialism, the self-styled scientific philosophy of Marxism.)

The fact is that 'free', 'compelled', 'active' and 'passive' are correlative terms. We cannot make sense of one term without presupposing the others. For this reason, to speak of 'absolute freedom' or 'absolute determinism' is nonsense. Similarly, to assert that there is a logical or empirical connection between factors or events which we label 'cause' and 'effect' does not mean, as Hume pointed out (Lindsay 1951), that the connection is either logically necessary or that some compulsion operates between 'cause' and 'effect', or that being able to predict (with a high degree of probability) what the result of some action may be forces the outcome.

The freedom required for moral action is the freedom of self-determination in a world where we have to choose between the various causal factors operative in a situation, understand our own limitations and the constraints placed on us by circumstances, environment or heredity, and by reflecting on the present situation confronting us, in the light of past experience, and, calculating the likely outcomes of various alternative courses of action, choose to become ourselves causes or determinants of other effects! (Downie 1971).

The questions to ask are perhaps those raised by Nietzsche (Cowan 1955) in commenting on the irrelevance of the free-will/determinism controversy to ethics (even though it might have entertainment value in metaphysics and theology):

Why should anyone want to delude themselves that they enjoy absolute freedom? Such a view is literally 'out of this world' and has more to do with individual will-to-power and delusions of grandeur than a responsible view of man's moral and political duty! Why should anyone want to maintain that all men are slaves to economic or material necessity? Unless their ulterior motive is to control people by encouraging them to abrogate their moral responsibility or to persuade oppressed people that they really are slaves and can do nothing to improve the world or their lot!

REFERENCES

Campbell A V, Higgs R 1982 In that case. Darton, Longman & Todd, London
Campbell A V 1984 Moral dilemmas in medicine, 2nd edn. Churchill Livingstone, Edinburgh, Ch2
Cowan M 1955 Nietzsche: Beyond good and evil. Henry Regnery, Chicago
Downie R S 1971 Roles and values. Methuen, London
Downie R S, Calman 1987 Healthy respect. Faber, London
Emmet D 1966 Rules, roles and relations. Macmillan, London
Hare R M 1952 The language of morals. Clarendon Press, Oxford
Lindsay A D (ed) 1951 Hume: A treatise on human nature, Vol 1, p 3. Dent, London
Nowell Smith P 1957 Ethics. Blackwell, Oxford
Pieper J 1959 Prudence: The first cardinal virtue. Faber, London
Roper N, Logan W, Tierney A 1981 Learning to use the nursing process. Churchill Livingstone, Edinburgh
Thompson I 1979 Dilemmas of dying: A study in the ethics of terminal care. Edinburgh University Press, Edinburgh
Thomson J A K (trans.) 1976 The ethics of Aristotle, revised edn. Penguin Books, Harmondsworth, bks 2,3,4
Toulmin S 1958 The place of reason in ethics. Cambridge University Press

10

The relevance of moral philosophy or ethical theory

10.1 Justifying our moral principles

In the previous chapters we discussed practical moral dilemmas in nursing in terms of the rights of patients and the duties of professionals, and discussed also the broader social responsibilities of nurses in terms of the principles of respect for persons, of beneficence and justice. In doing so, we have not questioned the concepts of rights and duty, and have taken for granted that what was said about respect for persons, beneficence and justice would be commonly understood. In other words we have taken for granted that there is a broad consensus in our society about the meaning of these fundamental moral concepts and principles. However, it must be obvious that we may question the basis of our belief in these concepts and principles. It is also obvious that some individuals within our society do not agree with the general moral consensus and, furthermore, that the form of moral consensus in other societies and cultures may differ from our own. To examine these questions is to engage in moral theory, and the systematic study of the means used to justify moral principles is what we call ethics, or moral philosophy.

The aim of this book is practical and therefore we have attempted to keep the amount of moral theory to a minimum.

Most stable societies have a long tradition of law and custom which embodies the established moral consensus of that society. Obviously, laws and customs do change and develop with time, and may change dramatically in times of war or revolution or rapid social change.

Recent public debate has focused on such issues as abortion, the rights of the mentally disordered, the definition of death, organ transplants, artificial insemination by donor, *in vitro* fertilisation and genetic engineering. The feelings aroused by these issues is evidence of the way new developments in medical science and technology challenge the established moral consensus, and people react to the demand to adapt or change their beliefs and attitudes to deal with the new moral issues raised by these developments. Social changes too, such as improvements in the economic and social status of women, earlier sexual development of teenagers, social migration and the impact of other cultures on our own, challenge (and perhaps threaten) settled moral attitudes and demand the negotiation of a new moral consensus.

However, social institutions cannot function without some stability in laws and customs. Some kind of moral consensus is necessary for the ordered functioning of society. In a relatively stable society we do not constantly question the moral consensus, and for all practical purposes do take it for granted in our day-to-day decision-making.

We do not normally question the basis of the existing moral consensus unless we are faced with a *crisis* of some sort. This may be a major social crisis or, less dramatically, a specific moral dilemma where we find our personal moral convictions at variance with what we are required to do, or where the majority viewpoint differs from our own. Here we are forced back to examine our first principles, to consider the kinds of reasons and evidence we would advance in defence of our moral principles.

Birth, copulation and death touch on our private lives most intimately, and these have traditionally been the areas most carefully hedged about with taboos to protect the rights and vulnerability of individuals. These are also the areas where modern society has challenged the traditional taboos most fundamentally and where modern technology has opened up whole new areas of ambiguity in the traditional moral consensus. Abortion and genetic engineering, fertility control and artificial insemination, euthanasia and suicide comprise a list of some of the controversies of modern moral debate both in medicine and the wider society.

If we are challenged to say why we think any of these things are wrong, or why we think they are morally justifiable, we may adopt one of a number of different strategies. We may say that we just 'feel' it is right or wrong, but do not really know why and would prefer not to discuss it. In so doing we may give expression to the view that moral beliefs are entirely private and subjective, that they are based on feeling or intuition and that moral disagreements cannot be settled by argument or appeal to evidence. Alternatively, we may argue that moral beliefs are decided by convention and that these differ from one society to the next. Different societies arrive at a consensus or some sort of social contract by reasoning together and agreeing to certain rules for their mutual protection and benefit. Other societies may have different kinds of conventions based on similar or different reasons and may or may not recognise the validity of one another's conventions. A third view may claim that there are and must be objective grounds for moral beliefs, otherwise they cannot be universally applicable and valid. From this point of view, the first leads to arbitrariness and irrationality, the second to relativism. Instead, it is argued, moral principles must be based on the way things are, the laws of moral behaviour must be grounded in the laws governing nature, the laws determining the physical and psychological well-being of man.

Moral principles, however we seek to justify them, are important for our day-to-day living and decision-making. They help in the ordering of moral experience and provide some sort of systematic basis for decision-making. They are both psychologically necessary to help make sense of our lives and moral experience, and practically useful in enabling us to make value judgements in a non-arbitrary manner. In both senses they assist us in our communication with others and in the rationalisation of co-operative action. It is because they perform this primitive ordering function of knowledge and action that we call them principles. It is doubtful whether anyone can do without principles in this sense, and continue to function in society.

Agreement about moral principles is obviously highly desirable and makes social life a lot easier and tidier. How do we
arrive at agreement, and what is meant by 'agreement'? The
view that moral principles are entirely private and subjective
is hard to maintain, if it means that they are arbitrary and
capricious. Such a view would lead to inconsistency in
individual practice and to anarchy in society. The fact is that
while we may agree to disagree about matters of taste, we *do*
dispute moral principles. That is because we recognise that
law and social institutions could not function without them,
and, in practice contracting into the moral consensus is a
condition of our being able and allowed to participate in
society. Underlying our continued and continuing arguments
is a conviction that moral principles must in some sense be
universal and objective. We continue to seek reasons and
evidence to establish moral agreement. We could take refuge
in irrationality but that is no defence — either for the sanctity
of our own moral beliefs or from the tyranny of those of
others. Reasoning together, trying to find rational grounds for
public agreement, is the way to establish moral principles as
universal (intersubjectively valid) and objective (grounded in
common human experience).

In whatever way we attempt to defend our moral principles
we are bound to one or other of these three strategies, or a
combination of them. The reason is that each strategy emphasises an aspect of moral experience important in itself. The
subjectivist is not traditionally concerned with the arbitrary
nature of moral judgements so much as to emphasise that we
do 'internalise' moral principles, make a personal commitment to them, make them our own and try to live our lives
in accordance with them. Moral principles are personal in this
sense, that they are believed and acted upon by persons who
may feel very strongly about them. This may, of course, introduce an element of bias or prejudice into their moral judgements, and people may not like to have these personal
feelings questioned or challenged. To the *conventionalist* the
most important fact to emphasise is the public and social
character of moral beliefs and their function as necessary
conditions for social intercourse and co-operation. Conven-
tionalists do tend to point out the variations in moral conventions between different societies, not primarily to stress the

relativity of all values, but rather to emphasise the need for tolerance of other people's values. The universality of moral principles can, in this view, only be established on the basis of negotiated rational agreement and tolerance of diversity. The *objectivist* is concerned to avoid the dangers of irrational subjectivism and a relativism which threatens to undermine the sense of moral obligation, the imperative character of moral principles. Objectivists seek to anchor the concepts of value and obligation in the real world and not in personal feeling or mere social convention. For them, moral principles must in some sense correspond to the demands of reality, as they believe the universality of moral principles and their objectivity can only be guaranteed in this way.

Plato suggested that there are three senses of 'agreement' relevant to moral agreement about principles (Hamilton 1960). The first sense is that there should be agreement between what a man believes and what he does, between what he practises and what he preaches. The second is that there should be agreement among all people that the principles they adopt will be universally binding on them. The third is that there should be agreement between moral principles and reality, between the moral law and the conditions which govern and make possible human life as we know it. These three senses of agreement correspond roughly to the three kinds of justification discussed, and perhaps we should recognise that while each sense emphasises an aspect of moral experience none is adequate by itself to cover the whole complex subject.

10.2 Varieties of moral theory

Many different kinds of theory have been put forward in the course of history to justify an existing moral consensus, or to justify particular moral principles. Many have been based on theological premises, others on historical, sociological or psychological theories. The following summary explores different kinds of logical justifications for moral principles. The ones we will discuss are, in historical order, natural law theory, agapeistic ethics, intuitionism, utilitarianism and deontological ethics. (For general reading on each type of theory see references at the end of the chapter.)

Natural Law theory

In its classical form it is difficult to disentangle this theory from traditional religious beliefs, in both the Graeco-Roman and Judeo-Christian traditions. In Sophocles' tragedy *Antigone* (Watling 1954), the eponymous heroine appeals against the tyranny, the arbitrary edict of the King which prohibits her from burying her brother. She appeals to the law of God, the universal justice, which governs the universe. The Stoics argued that the universe is rationally intelligible because it is a cosmos, that is, an ordered whole governed by rational laws. Human reason is just a part of the Divine Reason, the basis of this rational order in the universe, and that is why human reason can understand this order and should live in accordance with this given order in reality. In both cases the appeal to a moral law written into nature is, first, to resist the arbitrariness of personal edicts and the relativism of social conventions and, second, to explain the universality and interpersonal validity of moral principles.

When the Roman Empire expanded to include numerous other societies and cultures, Roman jurists found it necessary to develop a distinction between the conventional law of the societies they ruled (e.g. the Mosaic Law of the Jewish people) and the universal principles of law which they believed were applicable to all societies and by which the justice of conventional laws might be judged. The former was called the *jus gentium*, the latter the *jus naturale*. This jus naturale became the basis of what in the tradition of Roman–Dutch Law was called Natural Law. Two traditions developed in Roman–Dutch Law. The first emphasised the Stoics' view of the rationality of justice as being grounded in the rationality of the order of nature. The second, later tradition sought to ground the rationality of justice in the rationality of man and in the social contracts he develops to express that rationality. (See earlier discussion in Chapter 4.4)

The Roman Catholic tradition of law and morality has traditionally been based on a doctrine of Natural Law which tends to be reinforced by arguments taken from Revelation. In its classical form, the doctrine is similar to the Stoic one. It is argued that because God created the world an ordered whole, governed by laws, and man has the intelligence to grasp that fact, he can deduce from the observation of nature what it is necessary for him to do if he is to fulfil his human nature and live a fully human life in sociey with other men. In theory, that is all that we need presuppose if man is to deduce the laws necessary to avoid living an inhuman or subhuman life, or creating an inhumane society. In practice, the Natural Law is supplemented by appeal to Revelation — to the laws given to Moses and the teachings of Christ. When Catholics condemn contraception or abortion as evil, it is not always clear whether they do so on the basis of Natural Law or Biblical teaching, or a combination of both.

Historically, Natural Law theory in ethics and jurisprudence has had an enormous influence on the development of our social and legal institutions. When Americans seek to test the validity of laws by their consistency with the Constitution (which embodies a declaration of human rights), or when appeal is made to Common Law in England, appeal is being made to principles of justice which are considered more universal than statutory law. The United Nations Declaration of Human Rights, and other modern attempts to formulate universal human rights, make implicit or explicit appeal to the idea of rights as grounded in the nature of man as such, to Natural Law.

Agapeistic ethics

This unfamiliar phrase comes from agape, the Greek word for 'love', and refers to those ethical theories which seek to base moral principles and decision-making ultimately on love. The tradition stems chiefly from the Jewish and Christian religions, but is not confined to them. In contrast to the Natural Law tradition, which emphasises the rationality of man above everything else, the Judeo-Christian tradition seeks to define man's essential nature in terms of his capacity to love. In theological terms, the argument is that God is Love, and since man is made in the image of God the most important thing about man, the most important value in human life, is love. In terms of this theory, love is not only the ultimate test and justification for our moral principles, but it can also be the basis on which we make specific moral judgements, that is, by deciding what is the most loving thing to do in the circumstances.

Historically, agapeistic ethics developed in opposition to legalistic ethics based on religious and ritualistic taboos — whether these were believed to be of divine or human origin. At one level, agapeistic ethics is a protest against a conception of God as a god of stern justice insisting on ritual holiness. On the other hand, agapeistic ethics often takes the form of a protest against universal rules and laws, claiming that we cannot force concrete human situations in their everyday variety and uniqueness to fit the requirements of abstract general laws. Love demands recognition of the particular character of each unique human situation and the painful complexity of moral choices in real life. To live by love rather than by the demands of laws, it is claimed, is liberating, while living by law is restricting and guilt-inducing. Its critics argue that one cannot live without rules, that this antilaw (anti-nomian) attitude leads to anarchy.

In response to the charge of antinomianism, advocates of agapeistic ethics have adopted two different approaches. The first approach is to say that there is logic to our loves which does provide some guidelines as to how we should act. The second more radical alternative is to say that we do not need rules at all, that rules prejudge human situations and moral experience, that we must therefore approach each situation as far as possible without preconceptions and allow love to dictate to us what to do.

There are several examples of the first kind. The teachings of Saint Augustine are perhaps the most famous and most historically influential, those of Paul Ramsey (1980) perhaps the most important of recent theories. Saint Augustine argued that since God is Love and man is made in the image of God, then it is his capacity to love which characterises man's nature and it is achieving the right order of priority among his loves that constitutes the primary task of the moral life. But how do we know what is the right order? God has created nature as an ordered hierarchy of beings: from the physical elements to plants, insects, animals and man. (Saint Augustine would add angels at the top of the hierarchy.) Corresponding to this order in nature is an order in human life of the physical, emotional, intellectual and spiritual. Man's loves can be ordered in their moral importance accordingly. All other loves must be subordinated to *agape*. Love of God and love of fellowman, friendship, the desire for personal fulfilment, erotic love and basic physical appetite are each important in their own place, but unless each is subordinated to the other, in that order, then chaos results. Basic physical appetite must be subordinated to, and controlled by, the others or it leads to selfish exploitation of others and to one's own harm. The desire for self-fulfilment has to be subordinated to the demands of friendship and the higher duty to care for the well-being of others under God, and so on. Evil is deranged love, giving undue importance to lower loves over higher (Frankena 1964).

The second alternative, what has been called 'situation ethics' can also be traced to a saying of Saint Augustine: 'Love God, and do as you please.' However, in its modern form it owes more to the existentialist philosophers, particularly Jean-Paul Sartre and Albert Camus. Fletcher (1967), who attempted to apply this kind of love ethic to medicine, is of interest here. Broadly speaking, he argued that all the doctors and nurses need is their personal commitment to a love ethic and a sensitivity to what each human situation demands. Deciding what is right to do in each case means taking account of the unique circumstances of each patient, the nature of the caring relationship between health professional and patient. However, in dialogue with Paul Ramsey and William Frankena, Fletcher (1979) has somewhat qualified this simple position. What all three authors wrestle with is the tension between an ethic based on love which attempts to be faithful to the demands of the situation and the needs of the specific individual. Frankena (1964) and Ramsey (1983) both attempted to answer the need for rules in Christian ethics, as well as caring love or 'covenant love' (Ramsey's expression).

Intuitionism

While Natural Law theorists try to safeguard the objective and universal character of moral principles, and agapeistic theories emphasise personal commitment to values and the subjective element in moral judgement, both theories are complex and combine other elements as well. Both theories were historically rooted in belief in a God-made order, although secular forms have developed later which do not use the god hypothesis. Elements of convention come into both theories in their practical application.

Perhaps the purest form of subjective theory is intuitionism. It is the theory that we arrive at moral principles by rational introspection, by looking into our own minds and grasping what we find there. 'Intuition' means direct perception, insight. In popular terms, we know what is right by consulting our consciences. Intuitionism is the view that it is by direct inspection of our own minds that we know what to do.

Intuitionism comes in both simple and sophisticated forms, and perhaps there are elements of intuitionism in all ethical theories. For example, how in Natural Law theory one knows which elements of order are relevant to moral experience is a matter of moral insight. Similarly, knowing what is the most loving thing to do in a particular case means considering all the relevant factors and arriving at a judgement by some kind of intuition. At its crudest, intuitionism may represent a refusal to give reasons or evidence for a moral point of view, and retreat into inarticulate irrationality. But, more seriously, it is an attempt to draw attention to the activity of the moral subject as an essential factor in moral judgement. Computers cannot make moral judgements; it has to be a human subject, or moral agent, to do so.

Intuitionists have traditionally tried to avoid the charge that moral principles are the products of random, arbitrary and capricious judgement by arguing that there are given structures in the mind or moral experience which we intuit. For Plato, moral principles are in some sense innate. We are born with certain implicit moral ideas which it is the function of reason to make explicit in consciousness. For the early Quakers and certain Reformers, we know moral principles by illumination from the Divine Light or Holy Spirit. In defending the ultimate authority of personal conscience against the authority of the Church, they appealed to direct intuition of moral principles. For Kant, it is the introspective rational activity whereby we consider the principles which alone make reasoning and the rational life possible, that gives us insight into the form of the Moral Law. Intuition of what he called the *a priori* forms of reason is the ultimate basis on which we justify moral principles.

Intuitionism emphasises two important features of moral

experience: first, that our consciences are preformed in some way before we come to make moral judgements for ourselves and, second, that to be responsible moral agents we must have 'internalised' moral values and made them our own. We may explain the preformed character of conscience as did Plato, the Quakers or Kant, or we may explain conscience in terms of the process by which we are educated and socialised into the acceptance of a set of values. In practice, it is difficult to separate intuitionism from theories which explain the origin of moral principles in social convention. When someone says 'That is just not cricket', he appeals implicitly to the moral consensus among Englishmen as to what is acceptable behaviour and what is not. The 'intuition' of what is right or good tends to be filled out in practice by content drawn from religious tradition or social convention. However, as has been said, there is an element of personal judgement or intuition in the way moral principles are both understood and applied, and it is important that we recognise this.

Teleological or utilitarian theories

Teleological theories (Greek *telos*, end or purpose) seek to justify moral principles in terms of some overall goal or sense of purpose in nature or human society. Aristotle (320 BC), for example, argued that all living things have a built-in tendency to seek and grow towards their fulfilment. As the acorn tends to grow into an oak tree and reproduce itself by cross-fertilisation with other oak trees and so produce further acorns and oak trees, so animals strive towards the fulfilment or perfection of their form and reproduction of their kind. Man, in Aristotle's view, has a built-in tendency to strive towards his fulfilment, as a human being, of his physical, emotional and intellectual faculties. The goal which governs this striving is the pursuit of happiness, both in terms of personal well-being and fulfilment, and the happiness of the rest of society, since, he argues, man is a political animal and cannot be happy in isolation.

Aristotle's form of ethics has been described as teleological eudaemonism — 'teleological' because of his belief in the built-in purpose in nature, and 'eudaemonistic' because he saw human life as fundamentally motivated by the quest for

234 / *Nursing Ethics*

happiness, or well-being (from Greek *eudaimonia*). This system of ethics has been one of the most influential in the history of Western culture, and has greatly influenced Christian ethics, particularly in the Roman Catholic tradition.

Aristotle distinguished between 'pleasure' and 'happiness'. Whereas pleasure and pain are physical sensations or psychological states, happiness is a state of being. Pleasure and pain may be transitory and may relate to a part of the body or to particular feelings. Happiness, however, relates to the state of the whole person, is more enduring, and may persist even if the person is experiencing pain. Happiness, or well-being, is a disposition, or orientation, of a person's whole being and is thus directed towards some ultimate goal or ultimate good. Ethics as a whole is the ordering of life and life's priorities towards the achievement of this ultimate good and personal fulfilment. Virtue and vice are defined in terms of whether they promote or frustrate the achievement of personal and general social well-being.

In many respects, this theory has common elements with Natural Law theories, in emphasising that the tendency to strive for happiness is built into our nature as a law of our very being. It is not just a matter of subjective feeling or personal desire, but a given characteristic of human nature.

However, happiness can be interpreted as a desirable psychological state, rather than as a general state of being, and the striving towards happiness can be seen as a rational goal personally chosen, rather than something built in by nature. This interpretation of happiness was accepted by Epicurus (341–270BC) and his followers in antiquity, and by Jeremy Bentham and John Stuart Mill in the last century. Theories which interpret the pursuit of happiness as a chosen rational goal of human societies or individuals have been called *hedonist* (to the extent that the quest for pleasure and the avoidance of pain is the basis for making moral choices), or *utilitarian* (to the extent that actions or policies are assessed by their usefulness or practical value in adding to the sum total of human happiness).

The pursuit of pleasure as a principle for living can take both selfish and altruistic forms. The kind of hedonism associated with Epicurus and his followers was not self-indulgent, as common convention suggests, but concerned instead with a disciplined form of community life devoted to the higher intellectual pleasures and long-term 'happiness' rather than short-term carnal pleasures. Epicurus believed that man *ought* to pursue a life of pleasurable happiness and avoid pain, and that this could only be achieved by subordinating lower pleasures to higher ones, especially those of friendship. This kind of hedonism is called *moral hedonism* to distinguish it from *psychological hedonism* — the theory that human beings have no choice but are in fact always motivated by the instinct to seek pleasure and avoid pain.

Aristotle's theory has been called utilitarian, in so far as his test of the rightness of actions and moral principles is whether they are conducive to the greater good and happiness of men and society. However, his ethics was more tied to his biology and philosophy of nature, and his view was that the tendency to strive for happiness is inherent in man and not a matter of choice by individuals or agreed social policy. He would have agreed that man has to understand and strive consciously to achieve human fulfilment, but he would have argued that man also has a natural tendency to do so. Whereas the psychological hedonist considers man to be completely determined and unfree, Aristotle believed man to be capable of self-determination and thus of moral choice concerning his life and destiny.

Modern utilitarians are more concerned to emphasise the psychological nature of happiness — identifying it with feelings of pleasure and freedom from pain — and they stress that the pursuit of happiness, whether as an individual goal or social policy, is a matter of rational choice or social contract. At a simple everyday level the general utilitarian formula — choose the course of action which causes the least pain and maximises happiness for the greatest number — seems to be a useful guide to decision-making and dealing with moral dilemmas. However, when we look at the formula more critically it raises a number of questions. What do we mean by 'happiness'? How do we quantify 'pain' and 'pleasure'? Do we mean just those around us or the whole of society? Furthermore, when we attempt to apply the formula to specific actions are we talking about immediate psychological effects of our actions or the long-term costs and benefits to us and to society of utilitarianism as a policy for action?

Jeremy Bentham insisted that moral action consisted of obtaining *The maximum amount of happiness for the greatest number of people*. His attempt to provide a purely quantitative criterion runs into difficulties as soon as there is an attempt to apply it to actual calculations or discriminations between what are to count as 'pleasures' or 'pains'. Without qualitative moral criteria his hedonistic calculus proves of little practical application or to be based on arbitrary interpretations of the pleasure principle. While recognising the obvious defects of Bentham's formulation of the Greatest Happiness theory, John Stuart Mill also recognised its intuitive appeal as a practical test of the rightness of actions. He suggested several modifications which greatly strengthen the theory.

First, he recognised that we need qualitative moral criteria to distinguish between higher and lower pleasures, according to whether they serve the ultimate well-being of the individual. Second, he stressed the complexity of moral decisions, where the choice may not be between pleasure and pain but between different kinds of pains, or different kinds of pleasures: 'The principle of utility does not mean that any given pleasure, as music, for instance, or any given exemption from pain, as for example health, are to be looked upon as means to a collective something called happiness and to be derived on that account. They are desired and desirable in and for themselves; besides being a means, they are part of an end' (Lindsay). Third, Mill stressed that the things which count as contributing to the greatest happiness for the greatest number are to be measured by the criterion of greatest benefit to all. The shift from what Bentham called a 'felicific calculus' to cost/benefit analysis of the likely or actual consequences of actions in promoting the common good is what is definitive of his 'utilitarianism'.

The first modification introduces the principle of *totality* — the good of the whole rather than the part — to supplement the pleasure principle. The second suggests the need for some kind of *hierarchy* of pleasures, or qualitative criteria for prioritising pleasures, or for discriminating between desirable and undesirable pleasures. The third introduces covertly the concept of *good*, or benefit, combining both ultimate value to the individual and justice in terms of promoting the common good of society.

Modern philosophers have distinguished between *act utilitarianism* and *rule utilitarianism* (Frankena 1973). Bentham's simple formula, in so far as it is applied as a criterion to determine the rightness or wrongness of particular *acts* by considering their effects or consequence, and whether these obtain the maximum amount of happiness for the greatest number, could be taken as an example of act utilitarianism. On the basis of past experience it attempts to predict the likely outcomes of alternative courses of action, or it attempts to assess or evaluate the actual psychological consequences of actions already performed. Rule utilitarianism would judge an action right or wrong not according to its consequences in a particular case, but rather would judge an action right if it is based on a *rule*, following which it would be likely to lead to the best consequence for all. Mill's modified version of Bentham's General Happiness theory lends itself to interpretation as rule utilitarianism, since actions which serve the principle of totality, observe hierarchical distinctions between pleasures and serve the common good are not simply determined by attempts to measure degrees of pain or happiness. Rather, what is to count as 'happiness' or 'pain' is determined by one or other or all three of these additional rules.

Utilitarianism has an immediate appeal in health care since health professionals consider that they are in business to prevent or reduce pain where possible and to promote the health and well-being of patients. Because health professionals are expert at estimating what the likely consequences or side-effects of treatment may be, judging by consequences (act utilitarianism) appears scientific and reinforces their sense of authority in direct one-to-one clinical relationships. However, they feel less comfortable if asked to define 'health', 'quality of life' or 'happiness'. Similarly, when the nurse or doctor has to consider wider responsibilities to other patients, to the hospital, to the cause of nursing or medical research, to public health then rule utilitarianism is the more appealing — for health professionals often believe they know how the greatest benefit for the greatest number is to be achieved. However, defining 'justice' or 'the common good' is another matter, or justifying the connection between their clinical and moral authority. Campbell (1984) developed a strong argument for an historical link between the utilitarian tradition in Britain and the origins of the Welfare State, including the National Health Service. Be that as it may, attempts to sustain the Welfare State on utilitarian grounds alone (whether measured in terms of the costs and benefits of alternative forms of welfare provision, or the cost/effectiveness of different systems or practical services) raise fundamental questions about other non-utilitarian principles such as beneficence, justice and respect for personal rights.

Nevertheless, teleological and utilitarian theories emphasise certain important things about moral experience. First, goals are important in human life, whether they are conceived as built into our constitution as human beings, or chosen by us individually or on the basis of social agreement. Secondly, they emphasise that the practical application of principles and the consequences of actions have to be taken into account in determining whether they are right and good. Thirdly, the element of purposeful choice and the importance of the practical means chosen, are things to which these theories draw attention.

Deontological theories

The strongest criticism of teleological and utilitarian theories comes from deontological (Greek *deon*, duty) ethics. Kant, the most famous proponent of this theory, argued that it is not the end or consequences of an act which make it right or wrong but the moral intention of the agent. It is the good intention, the intention to do one's moral duty which determines whether an action is morally praiseworthy. To get to this view, Kant developed an argument about the nature of moral principles which has been of the greatest importance for ethics.

Kant maintained that for a moral principle to be binding as a duty, for a principle to be moral, it must be (a) universal, (b) unconditional and (c) imperative. He said we can never arrive at the notion of obligation from an empirical study of the tendencies built into nature, or from the psychological study of man's feelings about pleasure and pain. The concept of duty, he argues, follows as a logical consequence from our notion of rational practice. Human actions cannot be consistently *rational* unless they obey rules which are universal, unconditional and imperative.

In his *Groundwork to the metaphysics of morals*, Kant set out to analyse the principles presupposed in and necessary to the formulation of any coherent system of ethics (Paton 1969). His concern was to combat moral scepticism and relativism. Any system of ethics based purely on empirical observation of human nature or on the practical consequences of actions cannot lead to certainty but at best to probabilistic judgements. Alternatively, ethics based on feeling, risks being as arbitrary or fickle as capricious emotion. Unless moral duties are certain and absolute there is no way to gainsay the diversity of social mores and the apparent relativity of moral values. The way seems open to moral scepticism.

Kant's confidence in human reason and rational order in the universe was grounded partly in religious and metaphysical beliefs, partly in the logical proofs of his *Critique of Pure Reason* in which he had demonstrated to his satisfaction that without the *a priori* categories of pure reason we cannot make sense of the jumble of impressions we receive from our senses (Kemp-Smith 1973). Furthermore, he adduces from this given rationality in the world of our experience that this order must have its origin in a divine cosmic reason. In the *Critique of Practical Reason* Kant argued that there are three essential and necessary presuppositions of all morality, namely God, Freedom and Immortality (Beck 1949). God, in his terms, is a necessary postulate of morality, for without a god it would not be possible to ground the unconditional imperatives or absolute duties of the moral life. Without freedom or the power of self-determination and choice, we cannot speak of moral action or moral responsibility, as all we do would be automatic, reflex or conditioned behaviour. Kant considered immortality of the rational soul necessary to guarantee the transempirical validity of moral rules and the ultimate value of the life of man as a moral being.

In addition to these metaphysical arguments for the existence of God, human freedom of will and the immortality of the soul, Kant developed some powerful formal arguments about the essential logical requirements for an ethical system to be consistent and coherent. What he did was to explore what he called the constitutive and regulative principles of ethics as such. In more modern terms he set out to clarify the logical basis of ethics as a universe of discourse in its own right. If ethics is a way of speaking about the world and human actions in it, what are the rules of this 'language game'?

Kant adduced several concepts which are in his terms 'constitutive' of ethics as such: the concept of a moral law, the concept of a universal and coherent system of such laws, the concept of a person and the concept of a kingdom of ends. Kant was struck by the fact that moral duties are *not conditional* in form (If . . . then . . .) but *categorical* (Thou shalt. . ./I must do . . .). The moral 'ought', he argued, is categorical and imperative, but it is also, and must be, universal. Moral duties are not perceived to be binding unless they are understood to apply universally, to be binding on everyone. The concept of duty and universally binding moral laws follow logically, Kant believed, from the concept of a rational agent as such — a rational being who knows by rational introspection that he must act rationally in conformity with his own rational nature and the rational structure of the universe — if he is to live a life that is rationally self-consistent and thus satisfying to a rational being.

The concepts of 'personhood', and a 'rational kingdom of ends' are more substantive and less purely logical principles of an ethical system. As explained in Chapter 3 Section 5, Kant argued that ethics cannot get off the ground without the concept of a person, not merely as a rational agent, but as a bearer of rights and responsibilities. In the Groundwork, the definition of personhood he gives is abstract and formal. In order to apply the regulative principle of *respect for persons*, and, more specifically, to spell out what this means in terms of respect for particular human rights, requires that the 'blank cheque' has to be filled in with named attributes and the details of specific situations and 'transactions' before it can be 'cashed' in concrete terms. Similarly, behind his very abstract discussion of the principle of the universal kingdom of ends there is something like the principle of an all-embracing rational good or common end to which all rational beings are striving. And behind the principle of universalis-ability is the demand that the laws which apply to one should apply to all for the common good. Implicit in these two concepts is the principle of *justice*, or *universal fairness*. Finally, in the concept of duty and the principles of reciprocity ('Do as you would be done by') we come back to the principle of *beneficence*, the demand that we should care for other rational beings in order to assist one another to achieve fulfilment as moral and rational beings.

Deontological theories of ethics are often linked to religious beliefs and tend to be absolutist in form. The absolutist character of moral principles or duties can derive, as in Kant's case, from metaphysical and formal arguments about their logically necessary character, or they may be claimed to be absolute because commanded by God or based on sacred scriptures or pronounced by figures representing divine authority. Some kinds of Christian ethics are based on such absolutist deontological principles — exemplified by advocates of total pacifism, or 'pro-life' opponents of abortion or euthanasia under any circumstances — but Marxists and proponents of other secular ideologies may adopt similar stances on categorical duties.

Deontological theories have also taken two forms: *act deontology* and *rule deontology*. Act deontology is based on the claim to be able to intuit directly one's moral duty in a particular situation, by rational introspection. It represents a personal and subjective view of duty, and attempts to deter-mine whether particular actions are right or wrong on the basis of whether a person's motives were pure, or intentions were good and conformed to what an individual believed to be his duty. The appeal for Quakers of the Divine Light, or the appeal of the 'light of conscience', as well as some forms of rationalist belief in the illumination of rational intuition are variants of act deontology. As such, they are virtually indis-tinguishable from intuitionism and do not necessarily make claims about the universal validity or applicability of moral rules to all rational beings. By contrast, rule deontology is the position outlined earlier which tries to emphasise the universal, unconditional and imperative character of moral laws and moral duty. In this sense rule deontology attempts to establish that ethics has an objective, suprapersonal character, based on the universal rational structure of the universe and represented in microcosm in human reason. In terms of rule deontology, actions are right or wrong in so far as they conform to the universal, categorical and imperative character of moral rules within a coherent and consistent system of ethics.

The value of both forms of deontological ethics consists in the emphasis given to the notion of obligation as fundamental to ethics. Other systems of ethics in comparison may be said to fail to explain the sense of duty which transcends personal interest or possible pleasure or gain, exemplified by selfless service to others or personal sacrifice for a transcendent ideal. Absolutism has a prophetic quality in offering uncompromising opposition to what is seen as evil. While other more pragmatic approaches may seek compromise or may be vacillating and indecisive, an absolutist acts confidently and often courageously in the sincere conviction that he is right. However, absolutism may well lead to rigidity, intolerance and self-righteousness. In this sense, to adopt a phrase with apologies to Kant; absolutism without prudence is empty and formal, and worldly-wise prudence without principle is blind.

This criticism of empty formalism which is often levelled against deontological theories, and in particular Kant's, is both the strength and the weakness of this type of theory. Its strength lies in its universality and its emphasis on the suprapersonal, supranational character of moral laws. It is no accident that there is a direct line of connection between Kant, the later Idealists, and the principles which underlay the first attempts at world government in the League of Nations and the United Nations Declaration of Human Rights (UNO 1948). The weakness of the theory lies in the fact that the gap between the theoretical principles and their practical application is so wide that other lower-level concepts and principles are required to enable us to work with such ethics in practice. A related difficulty is that if we interpret all moral laws as universal and unconditional imperatives, then there is no way we can sensibly decide which rule to obey if we are faced with a conflict of duties (e.g. between telling the truth and protecting someone from a person who wishes to kill them). However, the abiding insight of deontological theory is that our ultimate (rather than derivative) moral principles must be universal and binding on us all if they are to serve as a basis for both individual and social life.

10.3 Moral theory and the structure of moral action

If it makes sense to analyse the process of moral and ordinary practical decision-making in terms of the stages of Assessment, Planning, Implementation and Evaluation (as in the Nursing Process and many other problem-solving methods), then it is perhaps not surprising to suggest that moral actions have a recognisable form or rational structure.

In classical and medieval thought, philosophers spoke of the intentional character of human acts in terms of the functional interdependence of agent and world in a teleological structure or purposeful set of relations between what they called *causes, means*, or *ends* (Maritain 1963). Causes in this analysis stood for both the objective conditions (or physical causes) prevailing or operative in a given situation and the subjective conditions (including professed principles and personal aims or motives) introduced by the agent. Means represented the alternative practical courses of action considered, the personal skills and physical resources available, and the particular set chosen to execute and action plan. Ends also did for the practical objectives or goals of the agent as subject, and the actual consequences or effects of an action.

Within this view of human and moral acts we have to take account of all three — causes, means and ends — in reaching a responsible decision, and if called upon to justify a particular action we should be able to do so after having made a proper assessment of the prevailing subjective and objective conditions, having made an informed and realistic plan based on available means and resources, and having anticipated correctly the likely consequences of the action taken to attain a goal.

The causes, means, ends structure of intentional acts suggests a model in terms of which sense can perhaps be made of some of the perennial disputes in moral philosophy between protagonists of different moral theories.

For example, protagonists of Natural Law theory (namely that moral laws are somehow grounded in nature) focus attention on the dimension of causes — the prevailing objective conditions in the circumstances of human action generally. Situation ethics (or the theory that we should act spontaneously in the light of the demands of the given situation) also interprets principles for action in terms of given circumstances. Intuitionism (or the theory which seeks to ground moral duty in pre-reflexive apprehension of moral principles) appeals to subjective reasons as motives or causes for action.

By contrast, pragmatism (the theory that something is right because it works) confines attention to means — to rational planning based on the calculation of available means and resources — to achieve aims. Existentialist ethics (Sartre: 'Man makes himself by his decisions') also stresses that in seeking to act morally man should not allow his actions to be predetermined by external causes or principles, nor influenced unduly by unpredictable consequences, but 'should act authentically in the given situation'.

Teleological theories of morals focus on ends. If, as in Plato and Aristotle, assumptions are made about nature itself and human action being ordered towards some ultimate goal or fulfilment, then the concept of 'end' is being interpreted at both a physical and a metaphysical level. At a more mundane level, utilitarianism grounds judgements of what is good or bad in terms of an assessment of the consequences or effects of an action, or of their general utility in promoting human happiness.

In a sense, what each of these types of theories does is to isolate one aspect of the intentional structure of human acts, and attempts to make it normative and definitive for the interpretation of all human action. The seemingly interminable debates among philosophers about the ultimate basis of moral judgements suggests that each of these theories may emphasise just one aspect of our moral experience. We may need to balance emphasis on one aspect with emphasis on other aspects of the whole causes/means/ends structure of moral acts (Downie & Calman 1987).

10.4 Moral theory and the goal of social consensus

The range and variety of theories developed to justify moral principles, the most important and abiding of which have been outlined above, may leave the impression that there can be no real moral agreement or that it is a matter of indifference which theory one chooses. This would be to misunderstand the kind of impulse which has led to the formulation of these theories.

What all these theories have in common is a belief that rational grounds for our moral principles can and must be found, that public agreement and objective decision-making in law and the moral life cannot be based on whim and arbitrary judgement. Each of the theories produces powerful arguments for the rationality of moral principles, whether we see the principles of respect for persons, justice and beneficence as being based on natural law, the demands of love, intuition, the requirements for the pursuit and achievement of happiness or the concept of duty. Each of these theories marshals certain kinds of evidence taken from moral experience and attempts to generalise its significance for an understanding of the nature of principles. It is tempting to say that each of these theories respresents a complementary aspect of moral experience and that, while each has some value, it is limited to the extent that it is generalised as a basis for the interpretation of all or every aspect of human moral life. However, there are some irreconcilable aspects of these theories and we cannot rest in such an embracing 'ecumenical' view.

We cannot do without rules or principles to organise our lives and moral experience. Society cannot function without some kind of moral consensus on which to base its social institutions. Law and order ultimately rest on government by consent, even under tyranny. No tyrant can succeed in isolation: he has to be able to persuade others to support his cause. The choice between might and right, between government by force and government by consent, if there is to be a choice, has to be based on reasoned argument. If we surrender our faith in reasoned argument, public debate and the possibility of social agreement, then we are lost to the forces of irrationalism, prejudice and anarchy. The only way to arrive at social consensus is by reasoning together — whether as a whole society or as a medical care team at ward level (Veatch 1981, Boyd et al 1986).

246 / *Nursing Ethics*

In practice, day-to-day decision-making does not involve discussion of this level of moral theory. We operate within the existing social consensus and do not question the basis of fundamental moral principles — unless challenged to do so. Perhaps the first time we begin to think critically about our moral beliefs is when we go to school and encounter people with different cultural or religious backgrounds. When we enter training for professional life we are introduced to a complex set of professional and institutional values which may challenge personal and moral beliefs based on family upbringing, education and conviction. When we encounter painful conflicts of duty in professional life (for example, between the duty to keep secrets and the duty to share information for the benefit of patients, or to choose between the rights of the mother and the father, or to preserve life or to alleviate pain) we are forced to examine the rational basis for our moral beliefs, and other people may demand that we justify them. When we move from junior to administrative responsibilities in large institutions we have to find criteria in terms of which to choose between the rules we use for dealing with individuals and the rules applicable to large groups of people. When we move out into public life — representing our colleagues in a union or taking part in local government or national politics — we have to begin to think through the connections between morality and law, ethics and politics. In all these situations, if we think critically and systematically about things, aspects of moral theory become relevant. We do not have to be philosophers to be concerned about these questions. We are drawn to think philosophically if we take seriously the quest for objectivity in ethical and legal debate, and this means adducing the best possible reasons and evidence we can for believing in moral principles at all. The moral theories we have outlined are only a guide to the way some great philosophers have thought about these questions in the past.

Reaching ultimate moral agreement may be an unobtainable goal but it is one of the grandest ambitions and most noble ideals of man. If it means agreement in the three senses we discussed earlier, agreement between what we profess and what we do, rational consensus or agreement among people about the principles of social life, and agreement between our principles and the demands of the inherent structures and dynamics of being, then moral agreement is a noble goal indeed. It is a symbol of a fully mature, fully human and genuinely humane society.

REFERENCES

Beck L W (trans.) 1949 Kant's Critique of practical reason and other writings in moral philosophy. Chicago university press, Chicago
Boyd K M, Callaghan B, Shotter E 1986 Life before death. SPCK, London, introduction
Campbell A V 1972 Moral Dilemmas in medicine. Churchill Livingstone, Edinburgh, Ch 3
Downie R S, Calman K 1987 Healthy respect. Faber, London, Chs 3, 4
Fletcher J 1967 Situation ethics. SCM Press, London
Fletcher J 1979 Humanhood: Essays in Biomedical ethics. Prometheus Books, New York
Frankena W K 1964 Love and principle in Christian ethics. In: Plantinga A (ed) Faith and philosophy. Eerdmans, Grand Rapids, Mich.
Frankena W K 1973 Ethics. Prentice Hall, Englewood Cliffs, N J
Hamilton W (trans.) 1960 Plato: Gorgias. Penguin Books, Harmondsworth
Kemp-Smith N (trans.) 1973 Immanuel Kant's Critique of pure reason. Macmillan, London
Lindsay A D (ed) 1910 Utilitarianism, liberty and representative government. Dent, London
Maritain J 1963 Moral Philosophy. Bles, London
Paton H J (trans) 1969 The Moral Law: Kant's Groundwork of the metaphysics of morals. Hutchinson, London
Ramsey P 1980 Basic christian ethics. University of Chicago Press, Chicago
Ramsey P 1983 Deeds and rules in Christian ethics, Univ of Amer. Press
Thomson J A K (trans) 1976 The ethics of Aristotle, revised edn. Penguin Books, Harmondsworth
Watling 1953 The Theban plays: Antigone, King Oedipus, Oedipus at Colonus, Penguin Books, Harmondsworth
UNO 1948 United Nations Declaration of Human Rights. United Nations Organization, New York. (Reproduced in: Campbell A V 1978 Medicine, Health and Justice. Churchill Livingstone, Edinburgh)
Veatch R M 1981 A theory of medical ethics. Basic Books, New York, Chs 4, 5

FURTHER READING

10.1 Justification of our moral principles

Hare R M 1952 The language of morals. Clarendon Press, Oxford, Ch 4
Toulmin S 1958 The place of reason in ethics, Cambridge University Press, Chs 11, 13–14

10.2 Varieties of moral theory

Natural Law theories

Cowen D V 1961 The Foundations of freedom. Oxford University Press
d'Entreves A P (1951) Natural Law: An introduction to legal philosophy.
    Hutchinson, London
Finnis J M 1980 Natural Law and natural rights. Oxford University Press
Wild J 1953 Plato's Modern enemies and the Theory of Natural Law.
    University of Chicago Press, Chicago

Agapeistic theories

Copleston F 1965 A history of philosophy, Vol 2, p 1. Doubleday, New
    York, Chs 7, 8
Gill R 1985 A textbook of Christian ethics. T & T Clark, Edinburgh,
    pp 135–152

Intuitionist ethics

Carritt E F 1928 Theory of morals. Oxford University Press
Moore G E 1962 Principia ethica, revised edn. Cambridge University Press,
    Chs 1, 3
Moore G E 1966 Ethics, 2nd edn. Oxford University Press
Broad C D 1930 Five types of ethical theory. Routledge & Kegan Paul,
    London

Teleological or utilitarian theories

Gillon R 1987 Philosophical medical ethics. Wiley, Chichester, Ch 4
Smart J J C, Williams B 1973 Utilitarianism for and against. Cambridge
    University Press

Deontological theories

Ross W D 1930 The right and the good. Oxford University Press
Ross D 1969 Kant's Ethical theory. Oxford University Press
Rumbold G 1986 Ethics in Nursing Practice. Baillière Tindall, London, Ch 5

General references on moral philosophy or ethical theory

Hare R M, 1981 Moral thinking: Its levels, methods and point. Oxford
    University Press
Macintyre A 1967 A short history of ethics. Routledge & Kegan Paul,
    London
Mackie J 1977 Ethics: Inventing right and wrong. Penguin Books,
    Harmondsworth
Raphael D D 1980 Moral philosophy. Oxford University Press.

Appendices

APPENDIX A: A PATIENT'S BILL OF RIGHTS

The American Hospital Association presents a Patient's Bill of Rights with the expectation that observance of these rights will contribute to more effective patient care and greater satisfaction for the patient, his physician, and the hospital organisation. Further, the Association presents these rights in the expectation that they will be supported by the hospital on behalf of its patients, as an integral part of the healing process. It is recognised that a personal relationship between the physician and the patient is essential for the provision of proper medical care. The traditional physician–patient relationship takes on a new dimension when care is rendered within an organisational structure. Legal precedent has established that the institution itself also has a responsibility to the patient. It is in recognition of these factors that these rights are affirmed.

1. The patient has the right to considerate and respectful care.

2. The patient has the right to obtain from his physician complete current information concerning his diagnosis, treatment and prognosis in terms the patient can be reasonably expected to understand. When it is not medically advisable to give such information to the patient, the information should be made available to an appropriate person on his behalf. He has the right to know, by name, the physician responsible for coordinating his care.

3. The patient has the right to receive from his physician information necessary to give informed consent prior to the start of any procedure and/or treatment. Except in emergencies, such information for informed consent should include but not necessarily be

limited to the specific procedure and/or treatment, the medically significant risks involved, and the probable duration of incapacitation. Where medically significant alternatives for care or treatment exist, or when the patient requests information concerning medical alternatives, the patient has the right to such information. The patient also has the right to know the name of the person responsible for the procedures and/or treatment.

4. The patient has the right to refuse treatment to the extent permitted by law and to be informed of the medical consequences of his action.

5. The patient has the right to every consideration of his privacy concerning his own medical care program. Case discussion, consultation, examination, and treatment are confidential and should be conducted discreetly. Those not directly involved in his care must have the permission of the patient to be present.

6. The patient has the right to expect that all communication and records pertaining to his care should be treated as confidential.

7. The patient has the right to expect that within its capacity a hospital must make reasonable response to the request of a patient for services. The hospital must provide evaluation, service, and/or referral as indicated by the urgency of the case. When medically permissible, a patient may be transferred to another facility only after he has received complete information and explanation concerning the needs for and alternative to such a transfer. The institution to which the patient is to be transferred must first have accepted the patient for transfer.

8. The patient has the right to obtain information as to any relationship of his hospital to other health care and educational institutions in so far as his care is concerned. The patient has the right to obtain information as to the existence of any professional relationships among individuals, by name, who are treating him.

9. The patient has the right to be advised if the hospital proposes to engage in or perform human experimentation affecting his care or treatment. The patient has the right to refuse to participate in such research projects.

10. The patient has the right to know in advance what appointment times and physicians are available and where. The patient has the right to expect that the hospital will provide a mechanism whereby he is informed by his physician or a delegate of the physician of the patient's continuing health care requirements following discharge.

11. The patient has the right to examine and receive an explanation of his bill regardless of source of payment.

12. The patient has the right to know what hospital rules and regulations apply to his conduct as a patient.

No catalogue of rights can guarantee for the patient the kind of treatment he has a right to expect. A hospital has many functions to perform, including the prevention and treatment of disease, the education of both health professionals and patients, and the conduct of clinical research. All these activities must be conducted with an overriding concern for the patient, and, above all, the recognition of his dignity as a human being. Success in achieving this recognition assures success in the defence of the rights of the patient.

(Reprinted with the permission of the American Hospital Association, copyright 1972)

APPENDIX B: HIPPOCRATIC OATH

I swear by Apollo the physician, by Aesculapius, Hygeia and Panacea, and I take to witness all the gods, all the goddesses, to keep according to my ability and my judgements the following Oath:

To consider dear to me as my parents him who taught me this art; to live in common with him and if necessary to share my goods with him; to look upon his children as my own brothers, to teach them this art if they so desire without fee or written promise; to impart to my sons and the sons of the master who taught me and the disciples who have enrolled themselves and have agreed to the rules of the profession, but to these alone, the precepts and the instruction. I will prescribe regimen for the good of my patients according to my ability and my judgement and never do harm to anyone. To please no one will I prescribe a deadly drug, nor give advice which may cause his death. Nor will I give a woman a pessary to procure abortion. But I will preserve the purity of my life and my art. I will not cut for stone, even for patients in whom the disease is manifest; I will leave this operation to be performed by practitioners (specialists in this art). In every house where I come I will enter only for the good of my patients, keeping myself far from all intentional ill-doing and all seduction, and especially from the pleasure of love with women or with men, be they free or slaves. All that may come to my knowledge in the exercise of my profession or outside of my profession or in daily commerce with men, which ought not to be spread abroad, I will keep secret and will never reveal. If I keep this oath faithfully, may I enjoy my life and practise my art, respected by all men and in all times; but if I swerve from it or violate it, may the reverse be my lot.

(Reprinted by permission: Dorland's American Illustrated Medical Dictionary, 25th edn. Saunders, Philadelphia, 1974)

APPENDIX C: DECLARATION OF GENEVA

Physician's Oath

At the time of being admitted as a member of the medical profession:

— I solemnly pledge myself to consecrate my life to the service of humanity;
— I will give to my teachers the respect and gratitude which is their due;
— I will practise my profession with conscience and dignity;
— the health of my patient will be my first consideration;
— I will maintain by all the means in my power, the honour and the noble traditions of the medical profession; my colleagues will be my brothers.

(Reprinted by permission: World Medical Association)

APPENDIX D: DECLARATION OF HELSINKI

Introduction

It is the mission of the medical doctor to safeguard the health of the people. His or her knowledge and conscience are dedicated to the fulfilment of this mission.

The Declaration of Geneva of the World Medical Association binds the doctor with the words, 'The health of my patient will be my first consideration,' And the International Code of Medical Ethics declares that, 'Any act or advice which could weaken physical or mental resistance of a human being may be used only in his interest.'

The purpose of biomedical research involving human subjects must be to improve diagnostic, therapeutic and prophylactic procedures and the understanding of the aetiology and pathogenesis of disease.

In current medical practice most diagnostic, therapeutic or prophylactic procedures involve hazards. This applies *a fortiori* to biomedical research. Medical progress is based on research which ultimately must rest in part on experimentation involving human subjects.

In the field of biomedical research a fundamental distinction must be recognised between medical research in which the aim is essentially diagnostic or therapeutic for a patient, and medical research, the essential object of which is purely scientific and without direct diagnostic or therapeutic value to the person subjected to the research.

Special caution must be exercised in the conduct of research which may affect the environment, and the welfare of animals used for research must be respected.

Because it is essential that the results of laboratory experiments be applied to human beings to further scientific knowledge and to help suffering humanity, the World Medical Association has prepared the following recommendations as a guide to every doctor in biomedical research involving human subjects. They should be kept under review in the future. It must be stressed that the standards as drafted are only a guide to physicians all over the world. Doctors are not relieved from criminal, civil and ethical responsibilities under the laws of their own countries.

I. Basic principles

1. Biomedical research involving human subjects must conform to generally accepted scientific principles and should be based on adequately performed laboratory and animal experimentation and on a thorough knowledge of the scientific literature.

2. The design and performance of each experimental procedure involving human subjects should be clearly formulated in an experimental protocol which should be transmitted to a specially appointed independent committee for consideration, comment and guidance.

3. Biomedical research involving human subjects should be conducted only by scientifically qualified persons and under the supervision of a clinically competent medical person. The responsibility for the human subject must always rest with a medically qualified person and never rest on the subject of the research, even though the subject has given his or her consent.

4. Biomedical research involving human subjects cannot legitimately be carried out unless the importance of the objective is in proportion to the inherent risk to the subject.

5. Every biomedical research project involving human subjects should be preceded by careful assessment of predictable risks in comparison with foreseeable benefits to the subject or to others. Concern for the interests of the subject must always prevail over the interests of science and society.

6. The right of the research subject to safeguard his or her integrity must always be respected. Every precaution should be taken to respect the privacy of the subject and to minimise the impact of the study on the subject's physical and mental integrity and on the personality of the subject.

7. Doctors should abstain from engaging in research projects involving human subjects unless they are satisfied that the hazards involved are believed to be predictable. Doctors should cease any investigation if the hazards are found to outweigh the potential benefits.

8. In publication of the results of his or her research, the doctor is obliged to preserve the accuracy of the results. Reports of experimentation not in accordance with the principles laid down in this Declaration should not be accepted for publication.

9. In any research on human beings, each potential subject must be adequately informed of the aims, methods, anticipated benefits and potential hazards of the study and the discomfort it may entail. He or she should be informed that he or she is at liberty to abstain from participation in the study and that he or she is free to withdraw his or her consent to participation at any time. The doctor should then obtain the subject's freely given informed consent, preferably in writing.

10. When obtaining informed consent for the research project the doctor should be particularly cautious if the subject is in a dependent relationship to him or her or may consent under duress. In that case the informed consent should be obtained by a doctor who is not engaged in the investigation and who is completely independent of this official relationship.

11. In the case of legal incompetence, informed consent should be obtained from the legal guardian in accordance with national legislation. Where physical or mental incapacity makes it impossible to obtain informed consent, or when the subject is a minor, permission from the responsible relative replaces that of the subject in accordance with national legislation.

12. The research protocol should always contain a statement of the ethical considerations involved and should indicate that the principles enunciated in the present Declaration are complied with.

II. Medical research combined with professional care (clinical research)

1. In the treatment of the sick person, the doctor must be free to use a new diagnostic and therapeutic measure, if in his or her judgement it offers hope of saving life, re-establishing health or alleviating suffering.

2. The potential benefits, hazards and discomfort of a new method should be weighed against the advantage of the best current diagnostic and therapeutic methods.

3. In any medical study, every patient — including those of a control group, if any — should be assured of the best proven diagnostic and therapeutic methods.

4. The refusal of the patient to participate in a study must never interfere with the doctor–patient relationship.

5. If the doctor considers it essential not to obtain informed consent, the specific reasons for this proposal should be stated in the experimental protocol for transmission to the independent committee.

6. The doctor can combine medical research with professional care, the objective being the acquisition of new medical knowledge, only to the extent that medical research is justified by its potential diagnostic or therapeutic value for the patient.

III. Non-therapeutic biomedical research involving human subjects (non-clinical biomedical research)

1. In the purely scientific application of medical research carried out on a human being, it is the duty of the doctor to remain the protector of the life and health of that person on whom biomedical research is being carried out.

2. The subjects should be volunteers — either healthy persons or patients for whom the experimental design is not related to the patient's illness.

3. The investigator or the investigating team should discontinue the research if in his/her or their judgement it may, if continued, be harmful to the individual.

4. In research on man, the interest of science and society should never take precedence over considerations related to the well-being of the subject.

(Adopted by the 18th World Medical Assembly, Helsinki, Finland, 1964, and revised by the 29th World Medical Assembly, Tokyo, Japan. 1975.) (Reprinted by permission: World Medical Association)

APPENDIX E: CODE FOR NURSES: ETHICAL CONCEPTS APPLIED TO NURSING

The fundamental responsibility of the nurse is fourfold: to promote health, to prevent illness, to restore health and to alleviate suffering. The need for nursing is universal. Inherent in nursing is respect for life, dignity and rights of man. It is unrestricted by considerations of nationality, race, creed, colour, age, sex, politics or social status. Nurses render health services to the individual, the family and the community and coordinate their services with those of related groups.

Nurses and people

The nurse's primary responsibility is to those people who require nursing care.

The nurse, in providing care, promotes an environment in which the values, customs and spiritual beliefs of the individual are respected.

The nurse holds in confidence personal information and uses judgement in sharing this information.

Nurses and practice

The nurse carries personal responsibility for nursing practice and for maintaining competence by continual learning.

The nurse maintains the highest standards of nursing care possible within the reality of a specific situation.

The nurse uses judgement in relation to individual competence when accepting and delegating responsibilities.

The nurse when acting in a professional capacity should at all times maintain standards of personal conduct which reflect credit upon the profession.

Nurses and society

The nurse shares with other citizens the responsibility for initiating and supporting action to meet the health and social needs of the public.

Nurses and co-workers

The nurse sustains a co-operative relationship with co-workers in nursing and other fields.

The nurse takes appropriate action to safeguard the individual when his care is endangered by a co-worker or any other person.

Nurses and the profession

The nurse plays the major role in determining and implementing desirable standards of nursing practice and nursing education.

The nurse is active in developing a core of professional knowledge.

The nurse, acting through the professional organisations, participates in establishing and maintaining equitable social and economic working conditions in nursing.

(Reprinted by permission: International Council of Nurses)

APPENDIX F: CODE OF PROFESSIONAL CONDUCT FOR THE NURSE, MIDWIFE AND HEALTH VISITOR

Each registered nurse, midwife and health visitor shall act, at all times, in such a manner as to justify public trust and confidence, to uphold and enhance the good standing and reputation of the profession, to serve the interests of society, and above all to safeguard the interests of individual patients and clients.

Each registered nurse, midwife and health visitor is accountable for his or her practice, and, in the exercise of professional accountability shall:

1. Act always in such a way as to promote and safeguard the well-being and interests of patients/clients;

2. Ensure that no action or omission on his/her part or within his/her sphere of influence is detrimental to the condition or safety of patients/clients;

3. Take every reasonable opportunity to maintain and improve professional knowledge and competence;

4. Acknowledge any limitations of competence and refuse in such cases to accept delegated functions without first having received instruction in regard to those functions and having been assessed as competent;

5. Work in a collaborative and co-operative manner with other health care professionals and recognise and respect their particular contributions within the health care team;

7. Make known to an appropriate person or authority any conscientious objection which may be relevant to professional practice;

8. Avoid any abuse of the privileged relationship which exists with patients/clients and of the privileged access allowed to their property, residence or workplace;

9. Respect confidential information obtained in the course of professional practice and refrain from disclosing such information without the consent of the patient/client, or a person entitled to act on his/her behalf, except where disclosure is required by law or by the order of a court or is necessary in the public interest;

10. Have regard to the environment of care and its physical, psychological and social effects on patients/clients, and also to the adequacy of resources, and make known to appropriate persons or authorities any circumstances which could place patients/clients in jeopardy or which militate against safe standards of practice;

11. Have regard to the workload of and the pressures on professional colleagues and subordinates and take appropriate action if these are seen to be such as to constitute abuse of the individual practitioner and/or to jeopardise safe standards of practice;

12. In the context of the individual's own knowledge, experience, and sphere of authority, assist peers and subordinates to develop professional competence in accordance with their needs;

13. Refuse to accept any gift, favour or hospitality which might be interpreted as seeking to exert undue influence to obtain preferential consideration;

14. Avoid the use of professional qualifications in the promotion of commercial products in order not to compromise the independence of professional judgement on which patients/clients rely.

(Reprinted by permission: United Kingdom Central Council for Nursing, Midwifery and Health Visiting. UKCC, 2nd edn, 1984)

APPENDIX G: CONFIDENTIALITY

E Summary of the principles on which to base professional judgement in matters of confidentiality.

1. That a patient/client has a right to expect that information given in confidence will be used only for the purpose for which it was given and will not be released to others without their consent.

2. That practitioners recognise the fundamental right of their patients/clients to have information about them held in secure and private storage.

3. That, where it is deemed appropriate to share information obtained in the course of professional practice with other health or social work practitioners, the practitioner who obtained the information must ensure, as far as is reasonable, before its release that it is being imparted in strict professional confidence and for a specific purpose.

4. That the responsibility to either disclose or withhold confidential information in the public interest lies with the individual practitioner, that he/she cannot delegate the decision, and that he/she cannot be required by a superior to disclose or withhold information against his/her will.

5. That a practitioner who chooses to breach the basic principle of confidentiality in the belief that it is necessary in the public interest must have considered the matter sufficiently to justify that decision.

6. That deliberate breaches of confidentiality other than with the consent of the patient/client should be exceptional.

(Reprinted by permission: United Kingdom Central Council for Nursing, Midwifery and Health Visiting. UKCC, 2nd edn, 1984. (Clause 9)

Author Index

259

Subject Index